My Clothes FIT *Again!*

My Clothes
FIT
Again!

The Overworked Women's
Guide to Losing Weight

Sue Seal

NEW YORK

LONDON • NASHVILLE • MELBOURNE • VANCOUVER

My Clothes FIT*Again!*
The Overworked Women's Guide to Losing Weight

Published in New York, New York, by Morgan James Publishing in partnership with Difference Press. Morgan James is a trademark of Morgan James, LLC. www.MorganJamesPublishing.com

ISBN 978-1-64279-954-5 paperback
ISBN 978-1-64279-955-2 eBook
ISBN 978-1-64279-956-9 Audio
Library of Congress Control Number: 2019919780

Cover Design Concept:
Jennifer Stimson

Editor:
Cory Hott

Cover Designer:
Rachel Lopez
www.r2cdesign.com

Book Coaching:
The Author Incubator

Interior Designer
Bonnie Bushman
The Whole Caboodle Graphic Design

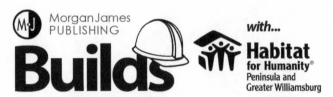

Morgan James is a proud partner of Habitat for Humanity Peninsula and Greater Williamsburg. Partners in building since 2006.

Get involved today! Visit
www.MorganJamesBuilds.com

To all the Superwomen of the world who give, love, perform, and serve beyond their need. To fit back into our clothes, we must strip our super suits. The mere act of saying "no" is saying "yes" to our future!
I love you!

Table of Contents

Chapter 1
Life Is Awesome, and Then It Is Challenging

"My life has been awesome and challenging, calm and hectic, happy and sad, rewarding and humbling, but in the space between those moments, I have learned to breathe and just be. And with my breath and myself, I have learned my life is mine."
– Sue Seal

"**W**hat do you want to be when you grow up?" the young boy asked his five-year-old friend.

"Nothing, I want to grow up to be nothing," she answered happily.

"What do you mean? You cannot grow up to be nothing. Why would you want that?"

"Because I always want to be as happy as I am right now," she answered before trotting off on her play stick horse.

One day, I think it just happens. We lose ourselves to life. It is not that we are unhappy—we just move so fast that sometimes we may forget to feel the joy life has to bring to us. We do not notice it at first because we are busy doing life. Life throws balls at us, and we juggle them in the air. Initially, as children, we have ourselves—we worry only about what we want and what we need, and we have only one ball that we are juggling. We can gently toss it in the air and catch it. It is super easy. Then, maybe we are challenged with a social event (a peer spat, or a fearful encounter—something social that causes us to worry or stress)—another ball to toss in the air. We strive for our profession or our career path—another ball. We start a relationship with a future mate—another ball. We purchase a house, and the financial worries place another ball in the air. We have a child, and another ball is tossed high. As women, we juggle, at minimum, six balls in the air.

I believe the first ball we drop is our self-ball. For whatever reason, subconsciously or consciously, we stop taking care of ourselves. Everyone comes before us. The weight gain starts the moment we cannot handle the balls we juggle in the air.

When we were children, we pretended that we would have this magical life when we grew up. Maybe we were going to be an astronaut, or the president, or a doctor, or a princess. It was always so enchanting and truly heartfelt. We played dress up and pretended to be a princess that lived in a castle or a doctor that had two houses. Maybe we married our prince charming, or became a famous actor. We had a beautiful family, and, of course, we would live happily ever after.

Somehow, I think we start with an image of who we will be and we strive to achieve it. Then, life happens, and we lose our selves, and we lose our body. We gain weight and lose our self-worth.

We have our children. We have our husbands. We have our houses and our jobs. But what I'm wondering is where did we go? When did we, as women, start to juggle all this? I see women juggling all the balls of life, and I feel that the woman is the center of the household in the family. She has strength beyond strength—a woman on a mission cannot be stopped. She will make whatever necessary happen if she believes it is her responsibility. When she has children, she wants their life to be perfect and flawless. She orchestrates her home and children as beautifully as she climbed the corporate ladder and managed her career.

As women, I believe we try so hard to make sure that everything runs smoothly. We tend to work the best when we can divide ourselves into so many little compartments. At work, we strive to be the best. We do the best we can, and we give with a compassionate heart. We typically succeed and grow to the top of the corporate ladder. We love our job and we are proud of it. We earn a lot of respect in our jobs.

Then, children come along, and we use that same pride, moxie, and determination to raise them. The thing about raising children is that it was what we were meant to do. We were put on this earth to have children, to raise the children and be the center of the home. Now, I'm excited about how far I've come in my life and how far women have come in our society. I am so proud of the female sex. We truly are amazing. If you look at every opportunity women participated in, we accomplished the duties extremely well and enriched it. I do believe that we work so hard, and are so successful at anything we attempt, but sometimes we forget a little bit about our own needs.

As we go through life, accomplish our profession, and have our children, we juggle two huge balls. We raise beautiful children, manage our house, and take care of the animals and all family members. We survive by doing. The weight crawls up—I know for myself that I didn't take the time to think about it.

Do you feel that you are too busy helping the children with their homework, making dinner, or doing the laundry to think about your needs? I bet you feel like you have jobs that never end. Do you feel like you are always racing? If you are like me, you feel like you never had time to think about yourself or took the time to think if that was good or bad. You took care of everyone, and I'm sure that's what you're doing right now.

Let's look at the typical day. You wake up in the morning and your children need help brushing their teeth and finding their clothes, book bags, and homework. You try to get ready for work, you pack up their bags, and make their lunch. You make sure they're wearing their socks—oh darn, where are their coats? They are in the laundry. You realize the coat is still in the washer and smells sour because you forgot to put it in the dryer last night. You discover the laundry wasn't done and feel as though it's consuming you. Then, you get to the breakfast, but who has time to cook anymore? You warm up a Costco muffin for the kids and yourself. You kiss the kids. "Have a great day," as you put them on the bus.

Time to brush your teeth and throw on your make-up. Half of the time, you put your make-up on in the car as you drive and eat your breakfast. I have one friend who told me, "One day, I'm going to be famous. I'm going to make one of these huge bibs that you can wear in the car so that we can eat our breakfast while we drive to our job." I must laugh at that. Just think about what we do and how we care for everyone else, and what we will do for ourselves is have a big bib on us as we drive in the car so we can multitask and not spill on our clothes.

I get you and how much you are doing. I am right there with you.

Let's continue your day at work. I remember one time in my career, about twenty years ago, at one of my first jobs as a physical therapist. I was just married. I visited my husband in another state on the weekends. One day, my employer came up to me and wanted me to head a huge project for the company that would need me to give up time on the weekends. He wanted to promote me. Of course, I felt great with the accolade, but I knew it would not be the right fit for my life at the time. He put pressure on me to accept the position.

Now, here is where we falter as women. Remember that we are the ones who keep everything together. We are the hub of the family, or the center of whatever we try to improve. Here is where we suck. We have a hard time saying no. I remember I told my employer (as he pushed and pushed me to accept a project), "I have enough on my plate currently and I am unable to perform that task right now. Maybe next quarter."

I get it—even if you say you can't do a task or a project, it still falls on your lap because we are unwilling to let things fail. Do you know what my employer said to me when I told him, "I have told you no. Why do you keep pushing me to say yes?" He said, and I quote, "You are a woman, and I know if I keep asking, you will do it."

We, as women, are encouraged to perform outrageous super tasks because we get the job done. We can do whatever we put our minds to. Now, sometimes—and I am as guilty as the next woman—it feels good to be so magical. I think we have superhuman potential. Am I right? I think this makes us feel a little bit better about ourselves, so we think, "Wow, I'm getting attention for this, so I'm going to do it because it makes me feel important."

Just before lunch, the cell phone rings—the kids forgot their uniforms for the soccer game. The homeroom teacher for your youngest asked you to help organize the field trip for the teachers' second-grade classroom. During our lunch, we jump in the car to take Johnny his uniform, and we call the PTA to share our outline of the field trip. That is what our lunch turns out to be, and then, after lunch, we get back into our professional roll, and we work as a team for the company. It is time to head home—oh my gosh. I don't know about you, but I didn't plan anything for dinner. On our way home, we realize the kids will be home and hungry. Fast food, baby. They love fast food, so I will get fast food.

Walking into the door, the kids come up to me and tell me about their day. They need help with their homework. The husband comes home and he doesn't have clothes to wear for work tomorrow—he reminds you that he might need clothes washed, so you throw in a second load after rewashing the coat from the morning. Then, you continue with your day: get the dishes done, homework is done, dogs need to be fed, and you know what? It is now 10:00 p.m. Where did the time go? Well, if you are like me, I just want five freaking minutes to call my own. I pour a glass of wine, grab some popcorn, and think I am going to watch a little TV. Within five minutes, I am asleep on the couch. Two hours later, I wake up on the couch with a stiff neck and stumble into bed.

The next morning, you repeat. Maybe the next morning you have a soccer game, or baseball game, or tennis match you must get the kids to. There is always something taking a little bit of your time.

What happened to us? When did we decide we could do it all or needed to do it all? I know when it was for me. That silly commercial, "I can bring home the bacon and fry it up in a pan…" I thought that was the coolest commercial ever when I was growing up. That was the beginning of our end as women. I just want to know, where did the women of the show Happy Days or Leave it to Beaver go? The only thing I ever saw June Cleaver doing on the show was sparkling a pan as the biggest job of her day. When did we take on the role of doing it all, being a superwoman?

With that being said, the weight just creeps up. We say, "What is happening to my body? I gain weight every day. I have no will power and I am so tired I can't even think about trying to diet. How did my body get so out of shape? It is as though in one night, my body just started to put on weight, and diets seem to make me fatter."

We do not have the time or energy to even look at ourselves, let alone take care of ourselves. I am not sure how many diets I tried, getting excited that this one is going to be the one that is going to work. It is exciting at first. You lose about ten pounds in the first two weeks—feeling great, jeans feel a little bit looser. Maybe you're still not in jeans, can't breathe well, and you still resort to wearing your spandex.

We continue this diet, and then—I don't know what happens—something happens to derail us from continuing the diet. I don't know if it's because we were not able to plan, or we were just too busy to eat correctly that day, but suddenly you feel sabotaged. The kids need something—they divert your attention away from yourself. It was a long work week, and you are just too tired to think of what foods will be okay on this diet you are on. There always seems to be something that creeps up on you that you need to give your attention to rather than yourself, and it is too stressful to continue with the diet. On those stressful days, the first thing I did was go to the cupboard, grab some Pringles, and pour a glass of wine. There goes the diet. "Dang it, I lost ten pounds—people even said I looked better. My self-esteem is in the toilet. Why did I even start this stupid diet anyway?" The next day, knowing that I blew it yesterday, I decide to give up on the diet. So, there goes another failed diet in my books. No more dieting for me—it was never going to work. I stop for dinner with the kids, since I don't have time to cook when I get home. I order a cheeseburger and three extra servings of fries. "Yeah, I'm going to have that dressing on my salad. Who cares? I blew the diet. What difference does it make?"

A couple of months go by—ten more pounds up. A new diet is all the rage. All your friends talk about it. You look at your coworker who lost sixty pounds on the paleo diet, or the keto diet, or whatever diet is in the news. Then, it happens again: you start; you do well; then, something happens; and, for some reason, it is sabotaged again.

I believe diets do not work. I believe we must understand exactly what is happening in our body, so we know what the food is doing to our body. It took me years to figure this out. Our bodies tell us what is good and bad for our system. The body will give us warning signs of what we need and what we're doing wrong.

The problem is, we stopped listening to our bodies.

When we were children, let's say, we fell and skinned our knees. We immediately stood up and one of our parents would say, "Brush it off. Keep moving." We were taught to ignore what our body was telling us. Our knee could be bleeding and rocks could be stuck in the skin, and we would brush it off and act as if it were no big deal. We learned to ignore symptoms that warn us that our bodies were out of balance. When we listen to our bodies, we uncover messages that will help us avoid weight gain and discomfort. Once we learn how to listen to our bodies and pay attention to what they are telling us, we will stop gaining the weight and be able to control the self-sabotaging, low-self-worth talk.

I believe diets do not work, and we no longer need to diet when we have a program that is functional and easy to achieve. I think once you understand what the body is trying to tell you and you understand, the weight will stay off naturally. For our bodies, we will be in balance and the weight will stay at our healthy place. We will feel energy because our bodies are getting fueled by what it needs to survive. The cravings will be gone. I learned how to listen to my body in order to take care of it. I want to teach you this same process. I want you to no longer feel tired, fat, and ugly. I want to help you enjoy every day, eating what you want and knowing what it will do for you or not.

I lost my weight, and I've kept it off for almost twenty years now. It never came back on. I learned what is harmful to my body and what my body needs for it to function at its best possible capacity.

Understanding what my body needs was key, but I also did a lot of different things to help myself understand my past. Later chapters will discuss triggers that we go through in life that possibly cause us to over-eat. We could have suffered from a trauma to our system—whether it is emotional, mental, or physical—that caused us to do certain things to cover up our pain. We will cover that in later chapters.

I've got you. I know exactly how you feel. I believe that we can uncover the reason for the weight gain and make it melt away. It did for me.

I want to help you stop feeling out of control with all your balls you juggle. I want to help you achieve that comfortable body that doesn't only need to live in spandex to be comfortable.

If I can do it, so can you.

I know what you feel, and I will share my story with you next. I have been there. I felt miserable, worthless, and shameful. If you are like me, you are just too busy working, raising children, and doing what you needed to do to survive. I thought, "What difference does it make if I worry about me?" It seemed selfish to think about me instead of everyone else. I got you. I know what to do to help you and give you some tips. Let me help you sort this out. I know I can help you make this time in your life become one of the best times in your life. If I can do it, you can do it.

Chapter 2
I Get You. I Was There.
This Is What I Know.

"Roma Sue, no one can take away your education. Learn as much as you can. For knowledge frees you to become your best."
– Derrell Homer Sharp

"You have gotten fat." He looked at me with his steel-blue eyes. "I know." I remember looking down at the bathroom floor. I looked back up at him and I said, "As soon as you are dead, I will take care of myself."

My father died one month later. I remember the day like it was yesterday. I was listening to Queen, "Get Down, Make Love." I couldn't play it as loudly as I wanted to. My mother took a black Sharpie marker two months prior and marked on the volume control the loudest I could play my music. My mom came in and said, "Your dad has died." I got up and went into the room, kissed his forehead, and said, "I hope where you are going, your life will be easier."

Back in my room, I didn't know what to do. We were in such shock six months ago when we found out he had cancer and was going to die. I looked at my watch. I had just enough time to jump on my ten-speed and make it to the school. Today was the day I was to take my driver education exam. I grabbed my backpack and walked out of the house. I started my life that day. I didn't mourn. I didn't look back.

Life seems to throw you curveballs, and then it gets easier. I was fifteen when my father died. I got extremely fat. I remember when it crept on. At first, my jeans were just a little tight. I thought I dried them too long in the dryer trying to get the wrinkles out of them. Then, one day, I had to lie down on the bed to zip them up. I learned that trick from my sisters. Jeans back in the day had not one stitch of stretch. They were like a vault: firm, binding, and awful. When I couldn't get the jeans to zip even while lying on the bed, I resorted to wearing overalls. I was going to make a fashion statement with them. I laughed and told everyone they would be the new style craze. That style didn't happen for another forty years until Mamma Mia came out and the beautiful Meryl Streep wore them in Greece. I continued to wear those overalls until one day I couldn't button the side of them. I decided then that I could just leave them unbuttoned. It wasn't until about a month later I couldn't fit into them.

I resorted to wearing a dress that had a crunchy elastic chest band, and then it ballooned out like a muumuu. I don't even remember where I got the dress. I think someone that came to visit Dad brought it for me. I was a little invisible in those days. There was so much going on in the house. I just wanted to quietly get through each day. I was responsible for making desserts, cleaning, laundry, and making more desserts. I loved this carrot cake and cream cheese frosting cake I made for the guests that came to visit Dad. I was alone in the kitchen, as always, and

I made up the cream cheese frosting. Of course, I had to taste it. Then, I had to taste it again. Soon, I had eaten the entire bowl of the frosting. I found myself doing that each time I made the carrot cake.

The funeral was upon us. My mom looked at me. "What are you wearing?" I was in the elastic chest dress. "Go and put something more presentable on." I turned away from her face and said, "I don't have anything else that fits."

Isn't that just how weight gain goes, though? One day, it is one of those easy days and you are breezing through your life. Life feels light and carefree. Then, there are other days that feel like you carry a massive weight around. The weight just sneaks up on you like a quiet fog. The thing I don't like—and maybe it is just me—is once you have been heavy or had a weight problem, every time you look in the mirror you still see that heavy person. You have this image in your mind that you are always heavy. I am not sure why, but that is what happened to me. I spent the next five years gaining weight and losing weight. I tried every diet there was just to lose weight and then gained it back.

I went off to college and I received my degree in physical therapy. I purchased my first house at age twenty-two. Once I bought this sweet house, I realized I now needed to buy a lawnmower. What the heck was I thinking buying a house at such a young age? I was a homeowner. I just jumped right into my life. I worked and worked and worked. The weight always seemed to sneak its way back on during those times when I was too busy to think about it: new jobs, promotions, and excelling in my profession.

At one time, I can remember thinking about my life as the year of "wine and roses." I planted a ton of roses in my backyard and I would walk through my yard every night enjoying them. I loved my job. It gave me a sense of accomplishment.

I started to have health problems. My stomach ached constantly. I had headaches and I suffered from endometriosis. I had surgery to remove scar tissue and a procedure to remove cancer growths on my cervix. My life just kept rolling along. Even though I suffered from health problems, I didn't stop to think about it. I was extremely happy at the time and felt somewhat invincible. I was promoted to a managerial position within two years of graduating. I was busy. I met and married my wonderful husband. We had five years of fun and freedom as a married couple climbing our corporate ladders. We decided that we wanted children after being married for about four years. I couldn't conceive.

It was at this time in my life when I tried to figure out what was going on with me.

In 1996, Oprah Winfrey had an enlightenment series with amazing guest speakers. Among them were Gary Zukav, John Gray, Christiane Northrup, and Maya Angelou, just to name a few.

One book that helped me to research the chakra system and learn more about my body was Christiane Northrup, MD's book, "Women's Bodies, Women's Wisdom: Creating Physical and Emotional Health and Healing." If you don't have this book, order it right now on Amazon. You will be so glad you did. I fully believe that, because of the Oprah series and Christiane's book, I was able to unlock my trauma that was preventing me from conceiving.

Christiane Northrup's book explained the chakras in-depth. What intrigued me was when one suffers from an emotional trauma of being abandoned at a young age due to a death of a loved one—the sacral chakra will become imbalanced. The sacral chakra is related to the reproductive organs.

I finally was blessed with two beautiful children. A little girl was our firstborn child—she had strawberry blonde curly hair—and we had a son, born three years after her.

I am not sure if this is how you feel. But the moment I had children, my life as I knew it stopped. My concerns and worries for myself stopped, and every ounce of my compassion went to making sure that my kids were happy. I think, as women, we somehow place a huge job on our hearts to be the one that makes everyone feel better. I know that I would drop anything I was doing to help my sad-eyed children overcome their issues, whether it was homework, peer drama, or whatever weighed their heart down.

I found myself lying awake at night worrying about what they went through. I no longer thought about what I went through. It was how I was going to help my children and my household be happy. The only time I was forced to think about myself was when I needed to get dressed for an event and none of my clothes fit. At that time, I felt so worthless. I wondered how this happened to me. It wasn't even the weight that was the worst. I got acne. I got cellulite all over my legs, and my arms got flabby. Worse yet, it got hard to keep up with the kids. Many times, they would ask me to play tag or race. I would make an excuse. I remember one day I thought to myself, "What is happening to me? I am tired, out of breath, and I can't move without pain."

I am sure by now you are wondering how I was able to stop my yo-yo dieting and weight management. Well, I stopped trying to diet. I know that sounds silly, but it is the truth

My profession as a physical therapist allowed me to understand how the physical body works: the joints, the fascia, the nervous system. For the first five years of my practice, I treated mainly the body. I would perform great manual therapy techniques and for some clients the symptoms would magically go away. Those were the times I felt as if I knew everything. Then, there were clients that just didn't do well. It didn't matter if it was the same area or same injury. Some clients would breeze through treatment and others would be stuck for months.

Here is an example of Beth and Sara. Names are not their actual names. Both clients were in a motor vehicle accident—rear-ended at approximately forty-five miles per hour. Both were about the same muscular build—Beth was a little leaner than Sarah. Both clients' x-rays and tests revealed mainly inflammation and no significant history of preexisting conditions. They were similar when they started therapy. Beth did extremely well with therapy, and within six weeks she was finished. Sara did not. The difference between Beth and Sara was that Beth was happy in her life. She was getting married and filled with Joy. Sara, on the other hand, was going through a divorce and hated her job. Sara was miserable in her life.

Sara was in fear each time she came to the clinic. She was in so much pain that she refused to move and perform the mobility exercises to help her regain the motion in her neck. Her body was in a constant state of inflammation. Regardless of what I tried nothing would reduce the inflammation she was suffering from. Sara took over six months to feel better, and then it wasn't that she wasn't 100 percent.

This baffled me. At that point, I realized that a person would heal faster if they were in a "good" place in their life. I watched several clients come and go, and some got better, and some didn't. I started to see a pattern. People who were in a state in their lives where they felt stressed or felt like life was taking control of them, they didn't do well. The people who were more in charge of their lives did well. I noticed that inflammation in the body would not go away if the client was overly stressed and in a sad place in their life. I noticed that fear, which was the driving force of the stress, caused some of my clients not to progress with their therapy.

As I continued with my professional career as a physical therapist, I noticed that many of the clients with different physical conditions in their body would feel better even though the physical condition remained. For example, for a person with disc degeneration, or osteoarthrosis, the degeneration in the body remained the same, but they would get better. Yet, some clients with the same physical anomalies— disc degeneration and osteoarthritis—would not do well at all. Digging deeper, I noticed that, invariably, when a client came to me under a lot of stress, if they were not in a good place in their life, they would have more inflammation in their body. Because of the inflammation, their body was slower to heal and actually sometimes would not respond to traditional conservative therapy. I needed to figure out a way to help the client reduce the systemic inflammation and, somehow, I realized that stress was the bottom of the body's inflammatory creator.

It was a little into my profession when I decided to mix Eastern and Western philosophies of medicine. I looked at the body and mind as a unit versus what the body only needed to heal. I studied a practice of Eastern methods of healing known as Jin Shin. It was developed years ago and is referred to as the mother of acupuncture. In this Eastern method of treatment, there are meridians that run through the body. Each meridian is associated with a body organ. There are depths in the meridians that are associated with emotions. In the eastern philosophy of illness, there is a belief that traumas can be stored in the body. Traumas can be physical, mental, or emotional. The body will store any of these traumas—whether it is physical, mental, or emotional—the same. For some of my clients who suffered from a physical trauma—let's say a car accident—they would have joint anomalies. However, if a client also had trauma from an emotional injury, they would have areas in their body that would be affected and hold onto the illness.

What I found in my practice is that if people suffered from a trauma, whether it was mental, physical, or emotional, they held it in their body, in the fascia or in the meridians, which set their body up for weight gain, illness or disease.

The Eastern philosophies of medical theory are briefly explained next. The life force of the person is composed of two forces: yin and yang. These forces travel along pathways in the body that are referred to as meridians.

The belief is that if the flow of energy becomes stagnate in the body along one of the meridians, illness or a disease in the body will occur.

Each meridian is either a yin or a yang. They pair together in balance; this pairing will cause a depth which is connected to an emotion. We have joy, anger, anxiety, pretense, grief, and fear/fright. I will take a closer look at the meridians later in the book. For now, it is important to realize that our body holds trauma in it. This was part of the missing link to why my clients did not get better.

The emotional response in our body at the different meridians are: The emotional components in the organs are as follows, the large intestine and the lung meridian are associated with grief, the small intestine and heart meridian are associated with pretense, the stomach and the spleen meridian are associated with worry and anxiety, the diaphragm and the umbilicus is our life force is associated with joy, the gallbladder and liver is associated with anger, the bladder and kidneys are associated with fear.

As I continued to progress with my career, I connected some of the emotions that people suffered from, which caused them to have a setback, and prevented them from getting better. I continue to mix Eastern and Western medicine. I studied yoga and became a certified Yoga Alliance instructor. I own my own yoga business, Balance Beyond the Mat. At this point in my career, I studied the chakra system further. I realized that chakras, when blocked prevent the body from developing into a healthy full functioning body.

In yoga, it is essential to connect the mind and body with the breath. I observed that postures and the way people carried themselves could be yet another block that held them back from health and weight loss. For example, a depressed posture with forward shoulders and head, and a slumped spine—this posture would be interrupted in the fascia as sadness or grief, which would impact the way the brain perceived the state of the person. More on this in later chapters.

There are seven chakras. Actually, there is a new belief that there are eight chakras. The eighth chakra is called the soul star chakra. It is your purpose in alignment with celestial purpose. This belief system works wonderfully with yoga and releases the fascia areas of restrictions and trauma held in the muscles and fascia lines. It also may help to find hidden messages that your body is telling you that, consciously, we are unable to bring forward to stop the self-sabotage of the diet dilemma.

The last piece of my career puzzle occurred when I looked at nutrition and how what we eat prevents us from health and weight loss. I realized there was something more that happened than just physical trauma to the body—mental and emotional trauma was also preventing full capacity to achieve optimal health. That physical trauma from food also affected the health and weight loss of my clients. Some of the food that we eat causes our bodies to have inflammation, illness, and disease.

Let's talk a little bit more about Sara. She came back for my help many years later. This time, she had gained over fifty pounds of weight and she wanted me to help her with weight loss. I have been working with Sara for about a year as a health coach. Sara is on a great self-awareness and weight loss path now. She hasn't yet reached her goals, but she is making amazing strides in health.

My approach to weight loss and improved functional health is looking at the mind and body as a unit, utilizing Eastern and Western philosophies to uncover underlying issues and to look at what we feed our bodies. How and what we eat, both for spirit and body, can help us achieve our weight and health goals or it can sabotage them.

I have developed a method that works. I combined all three of my career tools to create a method that not only looks at the foods that we eat as foods to fuel or body with nutrients—the actual food that we put in our mouths—but also the foundational foods that we use to fuel our mind, spirit, and soul with. The foundational foods are not actual foods we take into our mouth, but foods that feed our basic needs of survival.

In my program, I will help you uncover traumas that the body experienced, which are sometimes so hidden psychologically you may not even know you have traumas. These triggers could be causing eating binges or self-destructive behaviors.

My life has been amazing. I was fortunate to learn from my journey and rewrite some stories that didn't serve my purpose. I have my insecurities, faults, greatness, happy times, sad times, and anxious times. I had great parents that did the best they could with the knowledge they had. I have triggers that make my body and mind try to jump to a place of fear, sadness, anxiety, anger, and worry. I learned how to slow this process down, and that is what I want to share with you. My goal is to help as many women as I can to understand how truly wonderful they are.

How fantastic is my life? I get to help woman stop beating themselves up because of the weight that they can never seem to get rid of and love themselves as an amazing light in our world. I love that woman can get out of the spandex and into their fun clothes again.

---- ✘ ✘ ✘ ----

Chapter 3
Let's Do This

"Sometimes the bravest and most important thing you can do is just show up"

– Brené Brown

This is the plan we will use to get the weight off you. There are eight steps to my method. You need to do the steps in order.

I do like to use Eastern and Western philosophies of healing and understanding of the body in order to make this a simpler approach.

As I described in the previous chapters, I found that by combining the Eastern and Western philosophies, I can dig deeper into some of the reasons or the triggers that may cause you to gain weight. This process is fun and at no time should you feel the stress of trying to do everything all at once.

If you try to do too many steps at once, it will cause you to feel paralyzed and you will want to give up. Do not do this. I want you to realize that diets do not work. This is a lifestyle. You will learn what happens in your body and what your brain does with the foods that you feed it. We will look at the Eastern philosophies and address what some of your emotional blockages are by determining the state of your meridians and chakras. This all gives you an awareness of what your body does when we are stressed, fearful, or angry, and why sometimes we reach for unhealthy foods instead of eating healthier.

Step 1

The first step in my method is to find out a baseline of where you are in your life. I will, at this time, encourage you to grab a journal and start to write down your answers from my questions in the journal so you can refer to it.

This first step is about finding out where you are in your foundational food groups. Foundational food groups are our survival nutrition—what you feed your soul and spirit. This includes your relationships, your social life, your job, your home, your creativity or hobbies, your health, and your cooking. They include how you schedule yourself. Do you try to be a better person daily? How do you relax and have fun? The foundational foods are more of what we surround ourselves with. This is not talking about actual food that we are consuming for fuel. It is what we are experiencing in our day-to-day lives.

In this step, I will try to figure out where you are coming from. I will encourage you to perform some exercises that will take us through this process. One exercise is determining what you feed your foundational body or mind food. When I talk about foundational food, I am mainly talking about what you consume that is not food. For example, when you are in a relationship with your mate, that relationship feeds your heart and your brain, and it makes you feel good or bad, appreciated or underappreciated. This truly is an important food—if our relationships are degrading or emotionally troubling, it is like feeding our soul poison. I know that if you remember back to a time when you were falling in love, how wonderful you physically felt. That is because we release hormones that make us feel good when we are happy, and the opposite when we are sad.

The next item of your life I want to know a little bit about is your schedule. Think about what you do in the morning. When you get up, do you eat breakfast within an hour of rising? Do you give yourself a moment to think about your day? Look at hour to hour what you're doing during your day. Grab your journal and fill it out for that day with what you did through the day. When you rise, how long does it take you to get ready for work? Where and when do you eat? Do you sit down to eat, or do you try to eat while you do the laundry?

When were you the happiest in your lifetime? What music did you listen to? What were you doing for creativity, joy, and leisure? Were you in a relationship? What social activities did you enjoy?

How do you talk to yourself? I know this sounds silly, but it isn't silly at all. We will briefly go through the limbic system and the fight, flight and freeze also known as the sympathetic system in chapter four when we discuss stress. The autonomic nervous system can actually be stimulated even with the words we say to ourselves. Do you feel shame because of your weight? Do you criticize yourself for not getting enough done? Do you speak poorly to yourself when you're performing an activity? It is important for your brain to feel that you are happy with yourself.

Have you had any trauma? This is concerning trauma that is mental, physical or emotional. For example, mental trauma is worrying about your finances, your children, or getting to work on time. Are you worried about getting all your jobs done? Do you have mental trauma? Physical trauma refers to suffering from any illness. Was there physical trauma to your body in which a body part was injured? Maybe a car accident?

Chemical trauma is a form of physical trauma on the body and can occur from being on medicine or antibiotics for a long time.

Have you been under a stressful situation for long periods of time? Have you lost a loved one or suffered from a break-up or divorce? This would be an example of emotional trauma.

Traumas of the past that we sometimes try to bury can slowly cause disease in the body and turn into emotional triggers. Triggers for the past can be good or bad.

An emotional trigger for me was when I was nine years old. I was visiting with a man that was my father's friend. He was interested in talking to me. He wanted to know more about me. He wanted to know about my horse. He wanted to know about what I enjoyed doing and what activities I participated in, like the sports I liked to play. He was interested in me. I was so surprised that someone was interested in me. I felt happy. Right then, at that moment, I realized that I was truly happy. My father came around the corner and he said to me, "What the heck do you think you are, a gosh-darn ornament? Get in the house and get busy and help set the tables." I was devastated. That was a huge trigger in my life though. At that moment, I placed in my brain that myself worth and value was based on my efforts and work, not who I was as a person. My self-worth was centered around working hard, working for people, and performing jobs. It wasn't about who I was as a person. It's a trigger for me.

Another trigger can be a good trigger—your child gets attention from doing something extraordinary, for example. You recognize your child for their great achievements in math, or you recognize that your child is being fearless—all of those are triggers. The triggers will participate in the child's life in the future.

What are some of your memories that may have caused a trigger in your body? We will be talking a lot more about triggers in the later chapters of this book.

Step 2

Who do you want to be? Here we will go back through all your foundational food groups and decide who you want to be. What is the goal that you're trying to achieve? Without a destination, we will not achieve a goal. We will allow obstacles to stop us. Simon Sinek is a motivational speaker and organizational consultant that I was able to listen to. He spoke about having a destination and about achieving your destination. During the presentation, he asked an audience member to walk from one point of the room in a straight line to a spot in the corner of the room. He was specific about where he wanted them to go. As the person walked, he put a chair in front of her, and he told her to get to her destination. The person knew where she was supposed to go, so she just walked around the chair. But if Simon had not given her a specific destination of where he wanted the person to get to, the obstacle would have stopped her.

This is the same as trying to lose weight. This is important because this is your dream destination. What is your ideal picture of what you want to look like? Think about the person you want to be, not just the size or weight. How will it feel to walk, move in bed, and get in and out of your car? What makes you happy? Again, you're going to go over each of your foundational food groups and set a goal of where you want each one of them to be. This is where you will set your goals to your dream life.

Step 3

Determine what prevents you from achieving your dream life. In this section, I talk about your activities and how your foundational food groups may affect the success of your weight loss. I will also go over how stress affects your weight. We will discuss hormones and how stress affects those hormones. You will also learn about the choices that you make with your foundational food groups that might make you hold onto the weight. The timing of when you eat also plays a role in how we digest our food or set ourselves up for the day. We will analyze the actual food that you put in your mouth to fuel your body and determine if you make poor food choices.

Step 4

In the fourth step, we will look at what you feed your body more in-depth.

The food you fuel your body with. We've already talked about your foundational foods. I explained how important the foundational foods are and we will learn in chapter four, how this food group will affect your autonomic nervous system. When the autonomic nervous system is affected, we are either in stress and we release cortisol into our system or we are relaxed and allow our body to rest and digest our food. During stress, the blood will flow to your muscles for fight or flight. If we are stressed in our primary or our foundational food groups, we will not digest our food appropriately. This will cause us to gain weight. We will learn in this step about what you feed your body and what foods are good for you to eat. There are foods you should avoid because of how they are produced or changed in our country. The changes make it difficult for our body to process the food. I will also address serving sizes and how much to eat.

Step 5

Your body has a wonderful way of giving you hints in messages about how it feels. If the body shows different symptoms, these symptoms can be correlated to different parts of the body that are not functioning properly. We will look at different symptoms that you may have. This will include where the weight gain happens on your body. Different places where we gain weight can be due to hormonal imbalances. Digging deeper into your health, I will be looking at any past illnesses that may be contributing to weight gain. The gut can cause inflammation in our system, which could be destroying your health. In addition, we will address what the adrenal glands do and how they affect the hormones in your body. If you suffer from fatigue, there may be an imbalance contributing to your fatigue and weight gain. We will monitor your sleep look at your sleep cycles. For example, do you fall asleep quickly, do you stay asleep and get a full night's rest, or do you wake up in the middle of the night? What times do you wake up? We will be correlating them with Chinese Meridian time chart.

Step 6

It's time to detox. We will go through and detox your life. In the detox, we will not only detox your food, your gut, your sugar, and your liver, but we will also go over how to detox your house, the environment that you live in, people you surround yourself with, your pantry, your wi-fi, and what you cook with. We will even look at where you hold onto trauma in your body, to detox it. We will learn how to detox the fascia in our body with movement. We will add yoga, gentle stretching, and some high-intensity exercises to pump up the mitochondria in your body and to get rid of the ones that are weak. We will also detox the words that you say to yourself.

Step 7

At this point, you will be just about ready to ditch the spandex and be able to get back into your favorite clothes. It will be up to you to understand what you're doing in your life. If your foundational food groups are weak and are lower on the scale, they can be some of the reasons that you're gaining weight and not being able to lose the weight. More importantly, we need to figure out why they are low and why you push yourself so hard. Some of the lifestyle choices that you make may contribute to your weight gain and can be contributing to your unhealthiness.

Step 8

We will take our focus on not just losing the weight but gaining insight into better health. In this step, we will look at your attitude about your day, what you eat, and what you think. If you compare yourself when you look at other people, that affects you. We will go for the picture that you established. This is where we look at achieving the goals you set out to do in all areas of your life. We will look at how you will shift your life from doing to being. The body wants to be in balance, and in this step, you will complete the circle of going for the health in your life versus dieting.

I have completed a brief description of the steps that I developed in my program. Each of these steps allows you to understand your weight and health status a little bit better. As we learn what our body needs to perform at its most functional, optimal level, it will prompt us to provide it what it needs.

Chapter 4
I Want to Know You

*"You either walk inside your story and own it, or you stand outside
your story and hustle for your worthiness."*
– Brené Brown

Step 1

 t is time to look at our lives. I mean everything. I will ask you one
question, so answer it honestly. Do you suffer from stress? Even if
it is a small stress, if you feel it every day, it is a low-grade chronic
stress. In this chapter, I want to look at each one of your foundational
food groups and see how they serve your health.

Hey, while we are discussing stress, I would like to share what stress
does to your brain and body. But first, I would like to share some of the
areas of your brain that contribute to this weight gain and cause us to
stress out.

The Body on Stress

When we experience stress or we worry about something, we receive a message in our brain from a little place called the amygdala. The amygdala is an area in our brain that is the deciphering part of our brain. It is not where we use logic or our higher thought-processing centers. If the amygdala decides there is something we should feel threatened or worried about, it will notify an area of the brain called the hippocampus. The hippocampus and the amygdala form our limbic system in our brain, or the "emotional" portion of our brain.

The hippocampus is responsible for memory. The hippocampus takes short-term memory and turns it into long-term memory. More importantly, the hippocampus can correlate what we experience at present to something of the past. Sometimes, the limbic system has a little bit of bias on how it perceives the information. This is important, because it is how we have developed our responses to activities, emotions, and experiences. For example, if we experienced a childhood trauma of, say, someone calling us stupid during an activity, if there is a similar activity in the present time, the hippocampus remembers it and will connect those two activities. At that time, we feel those same emotions or the feelings that the experience made us feel when we were a child. We group the experiences. That fear or worry we experience will be grouped with some of our current experience, which makes our limbic system get a little bit hypersensitive.

Let's use a story of when I was rear-ended on the freeway. I have a memory tucked away in my body and in my brain. Normally, I wouldn't even remember the accident until it almost happens again. The near-accident experience causes my body and my brain to be stimulated to remember the episode. Now, let's say I am in traffic and a car comes up behind me super-fast. It will be at that exact moment that the amygdala will send a worry to the hippocampus. The hippocampus is a little hypersensitive about the past car accident—at that moment, it will immediately send a message to the hypothalamus. The hypothalamus in turn will send hormones to the pituitary gland in our body and to the adrenal glands in our body. When they are stimulated, they respond fast and it is like I have my foot on the hormonal gas pedal. Hormones flood the system, releasing cortisol and epinephrine. This occurs so we can move rapidly and get out of danger. Here's the tricky part—if the hippocampus remembers things from the past (my car accident), we become hypersensitive to stimuli that trigger emotional upsets or emotional happiness of the past.

The autonomic nervous system is now activated. There are two parts to this system. The first is sympathetic nervous system, which controls the fight, flight, or freeze response and releases cortisol and adrenaline. The second part of the autonomic nervous system is the parasympathetic system, which controls the rest and digest response. The autonomic nervous system is just what it says—it is automatic, it happens without our control. When the limbic system is on high alert, it will turn a worry into a fear. Fear will alert the autonomic nervous system, and it may be super sensitive to the emotion, and it will stimulate the sympathetic system. The sympathetic nervous system causes our blood to rush to the extremities; increases our heart rate, breathing, and blood pressure; and diverts the blood flow from our digestive system. Therefore, we stop digesting our foods.

I will analyze some of the triggers that cause us to go into fear. We will learn ways to stimulate the parasympathetic nervous system to perform rest and digest or stimulate our body to relax so we can digest our food. Can you begin to see how triggers from our past may cause us not to be logical when we are in distress? What about the constant stress of today's society and all the roles we juggle? We are in a state of chronic low-grade stress.

When we are constantly stimulating the stress hormones, not only do they get over-sensitized, but also when the limbic system is stimulated, it slows down the stimulation to the prefrontal cortex, which is where we perform higher thinking and use logic to figure out problems or situations. This causes us to have brain fog, anxiety, and depression. When the receptors are constantly stimulated for fear, our brain is hypersensitive to stimulation of the limbic system and the receptors become resistant to cortisol. This receptor resistance ignores all cortisol in our system. The excess in cortisol causes damage to the body in other areas. Unfortunately, it is like putting too much sugar in our body, as in insulin resistance. We will discuss this in length later in the book.

The Brain and Body Connection

One more important thought about the brain before we move on. There is a portion of the brain called the cingulate cortex that allows communication from the limbic system the "feelings" part of the brain to the prefrontal regions of the brain, or the "thinking" part of the brain. The anterior cingulate cortex notices all your mistakes. It remembers pain and it tends to dwell on the negative or what you're worried about. This portion of the brain tends to focus and put a lot of attention on what you see in front of you or what you're worried about or tend to think about a lot. For example, if you are constantly worried about speaking in public every time you go to speak in public, this part of your brain is stimulated for you to think more poorly about yourself. It keeps track of all the mistakes you have made. When you're nervous, the thought that you constantly believe or think to be true is brought to the forefront of your thoughts. Therefore, when we get so scared or worried, we ruminate on the negative. We need to re-train this area of our brain, and there are great ways to do this.

Imagine reprograming some of the wirings of all your mistakes that you constantly beat yourself up about. What if you were in control of the self-sabotage that we all do when we feel bad about ourselves? We tend to grab for the bag of chips or engage in quick eating. For now, one of the most important actions to do is try to replace the negative self-talk in your brain with something positive. This part of the brain is the reason we want to have a gratitude journal. If you look for positive or beautiful things around you, your brain will focus more on that.

Let's say you're driving to work, and maybe someone's been tailgating you. Instead of thinking about the tailgater and how they may hit your car, try to distract yourself. Give your brain a label to attach to. If you don't, your over sensitive brain will make you suddenly feel fear and stimulate the sympathetic system. The trigger from the past car accident has your brain super-charged to fear another accident. This will cause your body to respond with fear. If you distract your mind, but first take action physically and move your car so you're out of the way. Now, focus on something better—maybe a song on the radio, something that makes you happy, the blue sky, or the beautiful green trees. Focus on something positive. This will help reduce the pathways to this area of the brain that allows the emotional brain to run to fear and release cortisol. The brain is so amazing, and one of the things that we must realize about the brain is that it is an organ that can be trained. We can retrain the brain with a process called neuroplasticity.

There is another place in your brain called the dorsal striatum, which has two parts: an upper and lower part. The fun thing about the dorsal striatum is that the upper part is involved with your habits. For example, do you remember how hard it was initially to learn to tie your shoes? Well, the more you did it, the easier it became. Tying your shoe now is not even a thought—you just do it. The more you repeat your thoughts and actions, the more your brain will want to look for what you constantly look for. It will automatically look for that circuitry. For example, if you constantly look for the negative, that is pretty much all you're going to see. The brain is going to bring that to you. It wants to look for similarities that you like to look at. The brain says, "Hey, look, you know you're going to look for this negative item, so I will bring it to you." The brain will automatically look for negative objects versus positive objects. If you look for beauty, happiness, or goodwill, the brain will be more receptive to searching for good things to look at than bad. Looking for the positive will retrain the brain. The more that you look for positives, the more you increase the signals to the brain, which wants to label things fast. The brain will have a thicker pathway of circuitry for this emotion. It will look for something good instead of negative. It is the same area in the brain that makes you perform your habits. If you are sad, rejected, or happy and reach for a bag of chips or a glass of wine... guess what does this in your brain? The dorsal striatum, which is the section in your brain that remembers your habits and wants to make you fall back into the pattern that you use to self-soothe. Let's rewire this part of your brain with what your ideal life looks like.

Foundational Food Groups

The first step in our process is to find out where you are in your life. For our lives to feel complete, we have two sources of food groups that give us energy, movement, happiness, and life. The first and most important is the foundational food groups, or what you need for your soul and spirit to be fed. I will look at your foundational foods that feed your spirit. These are not actual foods that you eat, but what you need to survive in society. For example, your social relationships, your relationship with your mate, family, your career, your finances, et cetera. The foundational foods are what we surround ourselves with—they are the environment we place ourselves in. Secondly, we will discuss the actual foods you eat to give your physical body fuel.

Foundational food groups are what we need for our mind and spirit to survive in society. This area of nutrition for our body is not about food that we take in for fuel. It is about what feeds our soul, spirit, and life. It is our environmental factors that contribute to our development and our state of happiness. The chart can be found in the back of the book.

Relationships

The first foundational food group we will discuss is our relationship area. How is your relationship with your mate? Honestly score on a scale of one to ten how you feel right now with your mate. Do you feel appreciated, respected, and cared for? Can you speak openly to them, or do you feel like you need to hide certain information from them? If so, what do you hide? This could be a trigger from your past that we need to uncover. Do you feel listened to?

This area of your life, your relationship area with your mate, is a huge area of your time. You will spend most of your life with this person. When the children are gone, it's going to be you two together, alone without distractions. Some things to consider at this point—as I have witnessed over the past many years as a physical therapist and also as a health coach—is that sometimes, as women, we tend to place our children and their needs before our spouse. For me, when that happened, there was a little bit of distance in the relationship with my mate. Please also realize that I am not a relationship counselor. I am only trying to encourage you to review these areas in your life and possibly put some thought into them. If there is stress in this area, we will look at how this could affect your health and your weight gain.

Some helpful things to do with this if you did score lower than you would like: Try to schedule some of your time to cultivate this relationship. This exercise is mainly to assist you to uncover some areas that may need to be polished. If your relationship is a garden, picture it as beautiful rose garden. If you do not take time to weed and take care of the garden, the weeds will overtake the beautiful roses. We need to tend to our relationship with our mates, like we would tend to our beautiful garden. Pull the weeds. Give it some food.

Friends and Family/ Social Foundational Food Group

The next foundational food group that I want you to score is your friends and family. This is your social arena. Do you feel that you have someone who you could share your feelings with or have fun with? How you are with your social food is important. There have been studies performed that analyze the lives of people that are living past one hundred years of age. These areas have been referred to as the blue zones. The people lived a long healthy life in part because of their social connections. Studies have also shown a correlation that people that are isolated suffer from forms of depression and anxiety.

Who are the people who surround you? The people who you surround yourself with will impact our desires and achievements. Do you surround yourself with people who love you and want to see the best for you? Do the social groups who you surround yourself with build you up, encourage you to do better, pray for your prayers, and listen to you when you feel no one is there for you? Does your social group want to challenge you, meaning they make you want to be a better person?

Cherish this and hold them dear. If, however, your social network is not feeding your purpose—they are possibly competitive, or try to bring you down, if they do don't listen to your feelings, or they try to control you or stifle your growth. Worse yet, they are friends with you for the wrong reasons, for example, their desire to have you for their friend is solely for their own gains. This type of social network will only cause you illness.

This is an example of how a social situation can affect the brain and how we process some insecure feelings. Do you feel left out sometimes? The good old FOMO (fear of missing out)? This thought will stimulate a portion of your brain that says, "Hey, I told you that you were not popular or likable." That is the anterior cingulate cortex again. Now the hippocampus feels that this is a memory that is not good, so it relates it to a fearful time in your life. Once the hippocampus registers this as a negative experience, it then notifies the hypothalamus. The hypothalamus now will stimulate the fight, flight, or freeze system in your autonomic nervous system. Now, your body must release hormones to prepare itself for the danger. Once this part of your system is stimulated, the blood no longer goes to the digestive system. It goes to the muscles in order to give us the strength to get out of danger. Because of the memory of the fear that we were left out or excluded from our pack, your food will not be digested. It will be stored as fat since you are not able to digest your food.

Think about this example. You're home at night, and you're excited to be home to rest and enjoy your night, but you check out Snapchat or Facebook, and you realize that while you're at home, which is what you chose and wanted to do, you see that one of your best friends is out with another friend. Suddenly, you think, "Why didn't I get invited? Why didn't they call me? Well, gosh, they must not like me, or maybe I said something to them that made them mad." Here we go. This is the pattern that happens in our brain, and it doesn't make us feel any better. It makes us feel depressed. Did you realize that fifty percent of your feelings of loneliness are inherited from your parents' genetics? The other fifty percent is from your surroundings or the environment you place yourself in, both with your thoughts and with what you surround yourself with.

I must laugh at this because, if fifty percent of my emotions and my thought processes are from my parents' genetics, it isn't surprising I get nervous and have hard times. My mom was the twelfth of thirteen children and was born during the Great Depression.

Those times were tough—families had a difficult time surviving. A great movie that depicts the time was the movie Seabiscuit. The movie was set in the Great Depression. Families were no longer able to financially support their children. In the movie, they had to give their son away to another family because they could not afford to financially provide for him. Those were the times, I am sure, my mom wanted to always prove her worth to the family. We don't realize how much we are programmed from our genetics. However, we can change a lot of our programing by focusing on what we want to have in our lives. For example, if your parents were constant worriers, that could be something that you will be programed to do. If, however, you realize that this was something that your parents did, you can start to catch yourself and reprogram your brain. What I recommend when I start to worry is to look at the facts of the event I am worrying about. I stop saying, "What if?" I look at concrete facts. I also replace the worry with a positive thought. The brain will form pathways of circuits on what you think about the most. It wants to respond as quickly as it can to what you are thinking. If you start to look for the good things that may happen versus all the bad things, the pathway of circuitry in the brain will be stronger when looking for good.

My mom was born during the Depression. The family didn't have much money. My father became a prisoner of war for three and a half years. He had to take care of himself—people stole from him and he was on guard 24/7 for his life. No wonder I worry about stuff and think about what could happen, why things happen, or what I need to do to make sure I'm okay. I have done a lot of change for my brain, and now I have rewired it.

Back to the Facebook example. You are now worried that no one likes you. What you can do is label this thought. The brain wants a label to stop the swirling in the limbic system. Label it something like, "I wanted to stay home," or, "I was tired." The brain wants a fact. You probably told your friends that you were going to be home. When you decided to stay home for the night, you made a choice. You were happy with that choice until FOMO hit you. Now, once you see your friends out having fun, you start to second guess yourself. The brain will respond to this worry. Rather than predicting or guessing, clarify the fact to your brain. "I wanted to stay home. It has nothing to do with my friends not including me. It was my choice". The brain doesn't want you to predict. Predicting doesn't help anybody. Base your decisions on a fact, not a prediction or a feeling. If you feel lonesome, make sure to take care of yourself. Do something that you never have time to do. Pamper yourself.

How Do You Find Joy and Relax Foundational Food Group

Next, how do you relax? What creative outlet do you have? Do you find it necessary to have a glass of wine to unwind? What are your hobbies that entertain you? How do you relax at night? Do you collapse, or do you relax? Do you read, or do you watch TV? Do you engage in social media, and if so, how late are you looking at the blue screen?

How do you experience joy? What do you do with your downtime? I know, as mothers, our life tends to be going along with everyone else's schedule. I used to love painting. When the kids came along, I didn't have time to enjoy what I used to do. My time was taken up with their activities. When I struggled with weight, I never felt like I was having a downtime. I would finish my job and take care of the kids, the house, the farm, and everything else and collapse on the couch. I said I needed to watch TV to unwind, but I was asleep during the first commercial. I didn't know how to relax, have fun, or recharge. My go-to for relaxation was the enjoyment of a glass of wine.

At this point, it is important to respond to that time you were most happy. What activities, music, and hobbies did you do and enjoy? This is where we will rewire your brain. We will evaluate where you may be stuck in a loop as I was.

The Home: Another Foundational Food Group to Explore

Next, let's look at your home. This is a true gut-buster. Your home should be looked at as your friend. Do you treat your friend with respect, appreciation, and love? Is it cluttered or run down?

Is your home tidy or in disarray? Are there broken items in your home? Is it extremely clean? Think about where you are living and how your home makes you feel.

This is your cave. It provides shelter and protection for you. I encourage you to research Feng Shui. I read about Feng Shui when I was a little girl, about fourteen. I was trying to find safety in my environment. I realized that Eastern cultures build their homes in order to bring in health, wealth, and prosperity. Every room has a meaning, and according to how it faces—north, south, east or west—it can determine which areas of your home should be for health, family, prosperity and wealth.

Let's say you do not feel well. What if there is clutter or broken furniture in the area of your house that is for health? This can affect your health. Do you have broken furniture, lights burned out, clutter, or dirty objects? This could affect not only your energy but also your health. The belief in Eastern philosophies is that any time there is a block in the flow of the universal energy, like clutter or broken items, it can affect our health by slowing the energy that travels through our bodies. Now, in Western philosophies, we focus mainly on statistics and tests. The brain, if the clutter or broken items bother you, will once again stimulate our worry centers in the brain and our body will once again react. This feeling of clutter and dirt will stimulate—guess who?—our friend in the brain amygdala.

Your growth as a person foundational food group:

Next is your personal growth and learning, self-development foods that feed you.

How are you trying to be better? Do you run through life just trying to get by?

Our brain needs to be challenged to feel good, simple as that. When we stimulate the prefrontal cortex with good challenges, like a focused exercise or thought process, we decrease the negative emotions. Do you run from task to task? When was the last time you learned a new skill?

While I was growing up on a farm educational system, it wasn't the greatest. In second grade, my teacher asked me to stand in front of the class and spell shirt. Well, of course, I was nervous, and my autonomic nervous system was going crazy. My poor little prefrontal cortex had no chance to think logically. I sat there and spelled "S-H-I-T." Everyone laughed. I wanted to pee my pants. The teacher looked at me and said "S-H-I-R-T." I then realize my mistake. The reason for this quick story is because, at one part on my journey to where I am now, I volunteered at the elementary school second grade classroom. I thought it was fun, and I was able to participate in second grade all over again while helping the students. I still spell horribly, but at least I was able to challenge my brain. Rate yourself on your improvement. We need to challenge ourselves to learn and grow to keep our brain and body healthy. Do you try to be better every day?

Foundational Food Group of Cooking

The next area is about your cooking. Do you cook? Do you eat at home? Are you able to cook, or is your life schedule so busy that you're not able to cook? How do you feel about your cooking? Do you go to fast-food restaurants? How often do you eat out? Do you tend to eat the same thing over and over? What exactly are you cooking at your house?

When my weight was out of control, I was eating out at restaurants at least two, maybe three times a week. I was too tired to cook. I would go to work, pick up the kids, take them to their sporting events, finally get home about 7:00 p.m.—sometimes 10:00 p.m.—and I would try and figure out what to eat. Well, you can't have children wait that long, so we would stop at the fast-food restaurant, go through the drive-through, and grab something just to fill our tummies. We will go into this further in the next chapter about how terrible this is for your body, what we're truly eating from fast food restaurants. We will learn a lot about processed foods, sugar, and modified foods that we eat. Typically, when you go to a restaurant, their food choices are not whole foods or healthy foods. If you are home and you're able to cook, you bring out the creativity in you and that helps stimulate your brain for happiness.

Cooking also allows us to control what we feed our body. In Chapter 7, we will go over the foods that you eat, which give you nutrients for your body to use as fuel—real food. I'm talking about the real foods now, and at that point you will learn how the different types of food that we are eating and how it affects our microbiome, which is in our gut. The gut and the brain are connected, and they communicate with one another. If the microbiome wants certain foods, it will signal to the brain for you to crave it. Cooking is important: it allows you to control what you put in your body, which gives your body the fuel to move and function.

Movement Foundational Food Group.

How much are you exercising your gorgeous body: Another foundational food group is how much time you spend moving your body. Do you participate in some form of regular movement? If you do, what is it? Do you receive joy while doing it, or is it grueling? I know that we work hard, and we think that's enough physical activity. That is not the case. We need to have physical activity in which our heart rate increases and we move our body through patterns of movement. Without movement, our body becomes stiff, painful, and weak.

How are you moving your body? Do you think taking out the trash, cleaning the house, or watering your plants is a good enough cardiovascular fitness exercise? I have to laugh. I know when I was raising my children, I was exhausted just being a taxi mom, a tutor, a gardener, the cook, and the house cleaner. I thought I was working my body enough. Is that how you feel? We need to move our body so that it has some time to grow and heal and become stronger. We must have a sustained heart rate up for a time period. We need to move our joints through their full range of motion and perform some form of strengthening to keep our muscles strong so they don't shrink.

Our lungs need to be opened and used, and we must stretch that diaphragm so that we continue to have proper inhalation. There is only one way that you can connect your mind to your body: through your breath. When we breathe deeply with our diaphragm, we have more oxygen for our brain and our bodies. Many people breath from their accessory muscle in the neck. You can witness this by watching their chest and shoulders rise up and down. This form of breathing is not utilizing the diaphragm, which will become weak after not being used. When the body does not get enough air by fully expanding the diaphragm, your body becomes weak.

The horrible sad fact is that if we don't use our body, we do lose it. We lose strength, range of motion, balance, agility, and function. What do you do for movement? It needs to be something fun, not stressful, or guess what happens? We know the brain loop.

Your Career or Job Foundational Food Group

Does your profession or job fulfill you? Do you feel like you make a difference in the world? If this is the case, then we need to look at how much you have on your plate.

I wanted children and I wanted my profession. The mistake I made was not hiring help to help me manage the busy tasks of life. Please think about this for a moment. Women are the hub of our family. What we do is keep everyone on a level field. But if you make a difference in society and are raising our beautiful family, try to hire help. Hire a person that can manage the home and assume some of the tasks that can be performed by someone other than yourself. For example, the house cleaning, the taxi service for the children, and the day-to-day busy stuff that we can't stay on top of: laundry, shopping, housekeeping, and yard work. Hire someone to be a nanny to take your kids to their various activities. This is so important. The reason is because when you get home from your job you love that is making a difference to the world, your undivided time can be given to your family and your children. You will not be stretched beyond what is humanly capable. If you work and then come home to another full-time job as a homemaker, you will not be able to do either job well.

Analyze your career. Is it feeding you good, supportive food, or unhealthy food? You spend a lot of time in this area. Eight to ten hours a day, you are surrounded by this environment. Is it fun? Do you enjoy your work environment? Are you happy with your career? Do you feel like you're appreciated in your workplace? Do you get along with the people that are in your workplace? If you have chosen to be home, I respect that and honor you for that. The home manger is one of our most important careers for the future growth of our society. I realize that there is very little recognition and even less pay, but take this job seriously. Take pride in this, and realize you are making a difference raising respectable children for the future. You will also be providing a healthy environment for you, your mate and your children.

What you surround yourself with determines your biology. Make it amazing or change it to be amazing. Bruce Lipton, a cell biologist, wrote the book The Biology of Belief. As a cell biologist, he would study cells in a petri dish. The cells contained the same DNA structure, but he would change the medium or the environment in the petri dish. By changing the medium in the petri dish, it would changed the initial DNA cell structure into something new, it would build muscle tissue, bone, or skin depending on what environment was in the petri dish. What he realized and shared in his book is that we can impact our beliefs and biology by essentially rewriting or placing ourselves in a healthy, loving environment.

Is your environment at work a healthy one? Not only the career, but also the people who are nearest to you most of the day? If you work with a coworker who is angry and sad, this will impact you and your emotions. It isn't that the person is going to make you an angry person. They will bring your level of happiness down. We can pick up vibrational energies from other people. Our bodies feel the anger or bitterness of others, and it is sometimes difficult to ignore the heaviness they create. Who you surround yourself with, will contribute to how you feel and how your body functions.

Finances: Another Foundational Food Group

Next, we look at finances as part of our foundational foods. Believe it or not, finances do feed us emotionally, mentally, and physically. Are you stable and feeling comfortable, or are you nervous and worried about paying the bills?

Is money determining your life? Some people have so much money, but because of the amygdala, hippocampus, and memories of not having enough money from their past, the loop in their brain goes around and around. Money rules their emotions and self-worth. They allow their life to be ruled by money or material possession. Do you make enough money, but it isn't what you think is appropriate because of your past? Do you make enough but spend too much? Do you need more money to be safe? Either way, this impacts your health.

Foundational Food Group of Your Scheduled Time:

The next foundational food we need to look at is your schedule. When you wake up in the morning, do you rush out the door with no time to plan? Do you go from job to job and task to task without even thinking about your day? I want to introduce you to the Eastern philosophy of the Meridian clock. The meridians in our body are stronger at certain times of the day. If you align your day with the circadian rhythms, which are in alignment with the meridians in your body, the body will function better. If you can pattern your daily schedule close to the meridian clock, your health will improve, and you'll see better weight loss results.

Briefly, the traditional Chinese medicine body cycles starts at 6:00 a.m. to 8:00 a.m. with the large intestine meridian. The characteristics of this meridian, and to improve the flow of this meridian, is to arrive and to have breakfast and create balance.

Between 8:00 a.m. and 10:00 a.m. is the stomach meridian. The stomach meridians characteristic which will improve its natural flow and action are to make decisions, tackle task requiring concentration, and focus. At this time, it would be a good time to answer emails.

Between 10:00 a.m. and 12:00 p.m. is the spleen. The spleen meridians characteristics to improve flow are to perform joyful connections with each other. Connect with people and have soulful purpose or a nice lunch.

Between 12:00 p.m. and 2:00 p.m. is the heart meridian. The heart meridian characteristics to improve flow is to start slowing down. Slowing down brings clarity. Take a break in your day at this time. Breathe, and pause from the go to go schedule.

Between 2:00 p.m. and 4:00 p.m. is the small intestine meridian. The small intestines characteristics to improve the flow is for support. Schedule fewer intensive routines and tasks during this time, possibly schedule meetings with groups.

Between 4:00 p.m. and 6:00 p.m. is the bladder meridian. The bladder meridian characteristics for improved flow is it is time to wind down, have some social activity, and laugh.

Between 6:00 p.m. and 8:00 p.m. is the kidney meridian. The kidney meridian characteristics for improved flow would be to have dinner and be creative

Between 8:00 p.m. and 10:00 p.m. is the diaphragm meridian. The diaphragm meridian characteristics for improved flow is passage into rest, time to go to sleep to rest the body and the brain.

Between 10:00 p.m. and 12:00 a.m. is the umbilicus meridian. The umbilicus meridian characteristics to increase flow is to have courage and save conscious worrying of the day to day tasks to the higher unconscious states. As you sleep your brain continues to try to decipher your day to day thoughts and concerns, leave it to the unconscious to assist you with the problem. Have courage and allow for unconscious problem-solving.

Between 12:00 a.m. and 2:00 a.m. is the gallbladder meridian. The gallbladder meridian characteristics to improve flow is to allow the body and brain to receive recovery. Sleep and soul guidance are its perfect activities.

Between 2:00 a.m. and 4:00 a.m. is the liver meridian. The liver meridian characteristics to improve flow are sleep and inspiration.

Between 4:00 a.m. and 6:00 a.m. is the lung meridian. The lung meridian characteristics to improve flow is to progress to the waking state of the body, leaving the unconscious time of sleep. Wake up and bring on a new day.

It is interesting: If you follow that meridian clock, you slow yourself down.

Also, something I found in my practice that helps to determine possible blocked flow in one of the meridians, if you find yourself having reoccurring symptoms such as insomnia, headache, stomach aches, joint pain, at a certain repetitive time during the day, that meridian may be involved. It would be a good idea to look at the clock and correlate the time with that particular meridian. It could be a problem in that meridian.

Foundational Food Group of How You Talk to Yourself:

Now, I want to bring your focus to how you talk to yourself. What words do use when you talk to yourself? In the book *The Four Agreements* by Don Miguel Ruiz, the author explains how self-limiting beliefs may cause extra suffering and limitations in your life. The book is based on an ancient Toltec wisdom. One of the agreements is to use impeccable words. What you say to yourself, once again, the brain listens to. When you talk negatively about yourself or to yourself, it sends feedback to the autonomic nervous system. Once the autonomic nervous system stimulates the stress response, your digestion slows down. Do you say to yourself, "Oh my gosh I'm stupid," or do you say to yourself, "Oh gee, I missed that? I can get it next time."

Put a positive spin on your words. Stop criticizing yourself. It will help to increase the circuitry to be a more positive effect on the brain. Do you remember that old saying, "Sticks and stones may break my bones, but words will never hurt me?" That is so far from the truth. When we stimulate the autonomic nervous system with memories from fear, we release hormones that cause our body to have so much inflammation. With inflammation comes illness. We need to rephrase what we say. Instead of saying, "I can't afford that," say, "I chose to spend my money elsewhere." "I don't have any time"—rephrase it to say, "I have other activities that are more enjoyable." "I am so stressed out. I just can't get everything done"—rephrase it to, "I have an exciting and eventful life." Be careful what you say.

The body and your words have a vibrational frequency, and they will attract the same back to you. When you say you are so stressed out, you will perceive stress in every aspect of your life because your brain is looking for it to happen. Please be aware of what you say to your brain. If you say you can't do it, you will not be able to do it. Be careful with what you think and what you say. My brother used to tell me he was going to die as a young man. He died at age fifty-seven. My girlfriend suffered from breast cancer when she was young. She prayed that God would keep her alive until her kids graduated from school. She went into remission, but the cancer returned when her daughter graduated from college. She passed the year her daughter graduated. Words are powerful.

Your Foundational Food Group of Your Health

Another foundational food group that feeds our soul is your health. Do you feel like you're healthy? Just a little bit overweight, but regular health? No blood pressure problems? No diabetic problems? Allergies?

What illnesses have you suffered? Have you ever taken a long-time period of medications or antibiotics? Have you ever suffered from an infection? Have you ever been exposed to mold or metal? Have you ever had an illness that you could not shake? Was it a stomach flu or asthma? An infection? All of these can cause your body to hold onto weight.

Your health can be affected by your past childhood experiences. One last area to discuss is your childhood experiences. There was a study that was performed to determine if children who suffered from adverse childhoods would have a higher statistic to illness in their future. These experiences were called Adverse Childhood Experiences. For more information, visit http://www.cdc.gov/violenceprevention/acestudy/index.html

You can take the test below. This will rate your childhood experiences and give you a score. That score has been found to be in correlation to disease and illness in your later life. There are three types of ACEs:

1. Abuse: either physical, emotional, or sexual;
2. Neglect: either physical or emotional;
3. Household dysfunction: presence of mental illness in the family, mother treated violently, substance abuse, divorce, or incarcerated relative.

If you were in an environment where there was trauma, the ACE study will give you a number, and then we will see how this may affect your health.

This is just to make you aware of some factors that may encourage you to take a closer look at your body and try to adjust what you are doing in order to take care of yourself better. It is important for me to share with you that everybody goes through trauma. We will experience pain in our life. "Pain is inevitable, suffering is a choice," Buddha said. We will experience pain and trauma in our life, but the way we chose to handle it will determine our health. If we carry our trauma around like a trophy, cry, "Poor me," victimize ourselves, and let our trauma or our sadness define us, then we will suffer greatly, both emotionally and physically. If we allow our trauma to define us, we will be in a constant loop of self-destruction. Everybody experiences trauma. I am not trying to negate your trauma. If you did have a terrible childhood, it is up to you to not let it define who you are. It is a choice. The test can be found in the back of the book.

Chapter 5
A Picture Is Worth a Thousand Words

"You only have control over three things in your life-the thoughts you think, the images you visualize, and the actions you take."
– Jack Canfield

Step 2

To have a goal and a destination is the only way we will be successful. We looked at your foundational foods and we evaluated them. At this point, you can decide if you scored a ten on your foundational foods or closer to a zero. Have a goal in your mind of where you are heading. You can achieve this goal. Remember the Simon Sinek example? Have a destination and go towards it!

"No one saves us but ourselves. No one can, and no one may. We ourselves must walk the path."
– Buddha

About ten years ago, I read "Who Moved My Cheese? An Amazing Way to Deal with Change in Your Work and in Your Life" by Spencer Johnson. It was about mice in a maze. At one point in the maze, there was a great supply of cheese for the mice to eat. But, as luck would have it, the cheese supply stopped. There was no cheese for days. It was never coming back. One mouse thought that he would just sit there and feel sorry for himself and wait for the cheese to come back. The other mouse decided he wasn't going to just sit there and feel sorry for himself. He was going to find cheese. He decided that he was going to go for what he loved, and it was cheese. He left his home and went looking through this maze until he found his supply of cheese.

What I would like you to do at this point is have a vision of where you want to be—what you want your life to look like. I caution you about looking at models and magazines, or looking at only weight loss because, let's be real, the pictures in the magazines are all touched up, edited with photo tricks, wrinkle-reduced, fat-reduced, and cellulite-reduced. They aren't true. I want you to have a vision in your mind of what it would mean to you to be able to walk into your closet and pick out any outfit that you want. Let's take it a step further than just being able to put the clothes on. It is important, but I also want you to go back to your foundational foods. I want you to be able to walk into your closet and put your clothes on, but I also want you to be able to enjoy your social activities. The vision I would like you to look into is what body and image you place in your mind that will allow you to have great finances, a great house, the ability to cook, the ability to have a great relationship with your husband, and the ability to move your body and dance. What image is it going to be?

I will share with you what happened in my life. I cannot believe how powerful a picture is.

When I was graduating from college, I shared with you that I purchased a house. I was twenty-two years old. Prior to that little house, there was a vision that I had when, I believe, I was about ten years old. My brother and I pulled up to one of my dad's friend's house in Virginia. There was a twenty-four-feet-tall, rod iron gate that opened as we came to the driveway. When we got into the house, it was a beautiful, four-story brick mansion. It was a gorgeous place. My brother and I remember looking at each other. It was like, "We are not in Kansas anymore." This was a place and a lifestyle that we were not familiar with. The house was beautiful, of course, and the people that owned it were wealthy, but that wasn't what was important to me, it was how healthy they were. The next morning, I was trying to find the kitchen. I walked into this room in which Betty, the owner of the house, was sitting. She referred to the room as the green room. I stumbled into the green room and Betty was sitting in her rattan chair. She was dressed in a flowing white skirt and blouse, and she was holding a book up to eye level. I looked at the food that she was eating. She had lemon water sitting next to her, and she had a plate of fruit and cheese. This room was just gorgeous—it was all glass and there were tropical plants throughout it. I remember looking at Betty and thinking, "Wow, I don't think I've ever even seen my family read a book, let alone hold it up to your face or sit in a chair like that." My mouth was hanging open, and I was like, "What is this life?" To me, at that moment, I thought it was what happiness, wealth, and health looked like.

Back to after I graduated from school. I bought my house. I decided that I wanted a glass room like Betty. I had a glass room attached to my house. I made it happen because of the vision I had as a child. To me, every night sitting in that glass room reading a book was health, wealth, and happiness.

A picture is worth 1,000 words. Buddha says, 'What you think, you become."

The next picture I had in my mind at another point in my life was when I was told I could not have children. I went to the fertility clinic for five years, and the doctor said, "Well, physically, you should be able to get pregnant. I don't know what's happening to you." One night, I came across an advertisement for an SUV. The SUV advertisement had a Labrador dog sitting by the car and two children. There was a baseball bag and a bat, and then there was an equestrian saddle, boots, and a helmet. There were terracotta pots all sitting next to this SUV. What that SUV advertisement tried to say to me was you can have all of this in this car. I wasn't interested in the car. I wanted the lifestyle it showed. Flash forward, after I had my two kids, I did purchase an SUV, but what was cool was, as I was jumping off my back porch and running to the SUV, I saw my kids standing by the SUV. My daughter was going to equestrian lessons, and my son was going to baseball practice. In mid-jump, I looked at that, and there it was: the SUV advertisement, right there. The lab, our Daisy, was sitting by the SUV, my daughter was petting her ear, and she had her equestrian saddle sitting on the ground. Her boots were there. My son had his baseball bag and bat there. It was that picture: the picture that was in my mind. I made it come true.

After my mother died, I was in Hawaii, and I purchased another beautiful oil painting of water lilies. I fell in love with it. As a yoga instructor, I love water lilies and I love the lotus flower. I feel like we can all emerge from the deep, dark, murky water and come out shining bright and beautiful like the water lily. They sit in this muddy water, but they never have a spot of dirt and filth on them when they bloom. I didn't really have a place to put the painting in my house. I didn't have a wall big enough for it, so I decided to put it in my bedroom. Well, my husband and I decided to sell our farmhouse. We looked at so many houses, and with the market, some came and went quickly. The last house that I came to, I was walking up the entrance, and there was a Koi pond and all these beautiful lilies were in the koi pond. There were pink ones, white ones, and yellow ones, just like the painting. I knew that this is where I was supposed to be.

A picture is worth 1,000 words. What I want for you is to find a picture of the life you want to live. You can find a magazine advertisement that would give you the description of the life that you want.

The mind is powerful. Remember how I talked about the brain, and how when you don't decide, it is because you feel like you're going to fail? The brain wants to be able to label and control the environment if it can. Its prefrontal cortex does a great job of organizing things for you so that you can achieve and retain. This area of the brain is called the dorsal lateral prefrontal cortex. Its job is to mitigate the feelings of worry, anxiety, and fear and try to organize it. It allows you to focus on something else. The limbic system wants to worry, and it talks to the hippocampus. The hippocampus has the memory of the past. So, with that being said, if we don't have a goal, we worry.

Stress is produced in our body, and, once again, we can bring this all back to weight.

When the stress response happens because we are afraid to commit or are afraid to have a destination, our body and brain read that as stress. Our body looks and gets sick. When we worry, the limbic system talks to the hippocampus, and then the hippocampus is like, "Oh no, I remember this from the past week." The hippocampus has connected it to something wrong, which then stimulates the hypothalamus, which stimulates the autonomic nervous system, which, of course, causes fight or flight response. This all happens if you are in a chronic, low-grade stress life. If you're worried about something, you're not going to rest and digest your food.

So, now, let's go on a little bit about a study from the book The Talent Code: Greatness Isn't Born. It's Grown. by Daniel Coyle. This is an excellent book, and it analyses studies with the brain. In the book, it described one study in which they took children and had them practice piano for twenty minutes a day for seven days. The other a group of kids were told to practice the music in their minds. At the end of the study, the kids that didn't even get to touch the piano learned this new piece of music and were able to play it as well as the kids who played the piano physically. Nathan Tansharansky, a computer specialist who spent nine years in a USSR prison because he was accused of being a spy for the U.S., also demonstrated a similar case. While he was in solitary confinement, he played chess in his mind. He did it daily. When he got out of prison, he was able to beat the national chess champion.

It is your brain. It is so amazing. It is so beautiful. I have another really quick story about my daughter, when she was in her first neurobiology class. She had this brain in her hands. She looked up at her teacher and she said, "I'm holding someone's first love, first steps, first words, first memory. I'm holding someone's experience of their first math test in my hand." Most people don't think like this, or we don't realize what the brain does.

"To enjoy good health, to bring true happiness to one's family, to bring peace to all, one must first discipline and control one's mind. If a man can control his mind, he can find the way to enlightenment, and all wisdom and virtue will naturally come to him."
– Buddha

The next exercise that will be helpful in achieving your goals is to write down your goals and your destination as if you're living it right now. In this exercise, you will get the journal and write down everything you want to gain in your life. Write as if you are already living the dream. What are you wearing? Who are you with? How do your clothes fit? How are you making choices about what you're eating? How does your skin look? How do you feel when you stand up? How does it feel when you run up the steps? Imagine that you already achieved it. Because, once again, we're putting this out to the universe. You're setting your intentions.

Now, I'm going to walk you through what your picture needs to include. Go back and we will put your career in your picture. If you can find a picture that would represent how you feel with your career, how you would feel with your finances, what exactly would you want to be able to do with your money? Would you want to be able to save for a college fund for your kids? Would you want to be able to purchase a house? Would you just be happy living where you are and not worrying about bills?

With each one of your foundational food groups, you will give yourself a dream picture of a ten. Go through them all: career, education, self-help, and your health. Do you what you want to do to improve yourself. What areas do you feel that you want to excel in? Stand in your integrity, be a better person, have a dream, and be the image.

Physical activity, movement, and—you know the dreaded word—exercise! I prefer to say movement. Get your body moving. Dance, hike, walk, swim—any form of movement will help your body maintain its function. Instead of saying, "I want to be able to fit into my jeans," what activity would you like to do that you don't think that you can do, but you've always wanted to. Maybe it is to climb a mountain or swim across the lake. Would it be riding a horse? Would it be to run a marathon? Write it down.

The next foundational food is of your home. What does it look like when you walk into it? What do the rooms in your home look like? The last exercise now will be about your energy in your house.

More recently, I read another great book on the subject, *The Happy Home: Your Guide to Creating a Happy, Healthy, Wealthy Life* by Patricia Lohan. The front door of your house is the mouth and that is where the energy comes in, through the front door. The windows are the eyes. The walls are its ears. It is important that the energy in the house is free to flow. What causes the energy to become stagnant and slow the flow are broken items, uncomfortable couches, and clutter lying around. It is important that for you to have the house that you're living in. Your friend, the house, is considered with respect. Your friend should be allowed to have energy that flows through the house so that nothing becomes stagnant. Make sure that there are no cobwebs, dirty windows, or broken doors. If your front door is broken, this slows energy from coming into your life. You want the energy to flow through your house.

Next, look at the relationships in your life. Picture what you want the people in your life to look like. There may be some relationships that may not be serving you to become a better person. If those relationships make you unhealthy, place the type of relationship you want in your dream journal. What would be the best relationship that you could have with a friend? How could it improve?

The relationships with your husband or your lover, how do they look? The picture and journal is yours to have. What do you want—remember, we need to have a destination.

What is the dream social life you want? Are there people in your life who may drag you down? If, in this area of your social life, you found that you scored a little low, now picture your social life exactly how you would like it. When I did this goal, I said, "I will have two social events at my house per month. I will engage myself in a social activity at least once a week with my group that feeds my soul."

Spirituality: this one's a big one. It doesn't matter what you believe in—it could be the universe, God, or whatever your higher forces are for you. It may be nature. Try to connect with it. If it's nature, picture yourself taking more hikes. If it is the universe, connect with it. If it's God, talk to Him.

There were studies that show that when elderly people do not have a hobby, they get depressed. Our brain needs to be working on something. It needs to have a focus, even if the focus is painting a picture, doing woodworking projects, or gardening. What will your creative outlet be?

Picture your health how you want it to be. Right now, you struggle with weight. Are there other areas in your body and your mind that you feel like aren't just right? Do you have high blood pressure? Do you have asthma? What is the picture of health for you? Have a picture in your mind or find one. For me, I was lucky to be able to have pictures that had a meaning, like the picture of Betty sitting in that chair in that beautiful environment. To me, that was a picture of health, happiness, and wealth, so I made that happen for myself. The next picture for me was when I could not have children. It was a picture that represented an entire life. It wasn't just an object. The last picture that was important in my life was the lilies coming out of the mud in this beautiful oil painting. I ended up buying my house, and the entrance of the house has a koi pond with water lilies.

When we make a decision or a goal, what happens in our brain is the prefrontal cortex is able to shut down some of the old memories from the hippocampus. It helps us to have control over our future and our current life versus being held in the past.

---- * ✖ * ----

Chapter 6
What Prevents You from Your Dream Body

"Your life isn't about a big break. It's about taking one significant life-transforming step at a time."

– Oprah

Step 3

What prevents you from your dream body in life now? In Step 2, we established a goal of what you wanted your life and your what your body looked like. We did picture visualization and we gave our brain a destination. Now, there are times we dieted, and we've lost weight. We felt great, and then, suddenly, we go off the diet and gain the weight back. For some reason, we can't figure out why that is happening. I bet you think it's all about willpower, that you're not strong enough to stay on a diet, or that you give up, or that you're not organized enough to stay on a diet. For some reason, you give up the diet and you gain the weight back. I bet you think it's all about your willpower, right? I'm going to tell you that is wrong. It's not about willpower. Humans have great willpower. What happens is previous triggers from the past—gut dys-biosis, hormone imbalance, and or trauma—are held in the body, causing us to stop trying to stay on the diet.

Let's examine what happens that prevents you from getting the desired body. In this chapter, we will be going over hormones, the gut, and how stress affects weight gain. We will be addressing past triggers that may cause us to reach for the food for comfort. We will also be addressing sugar imbalances, which cause the gut to go into this dys-biosis, which means not in balance.

As I've said in the past, the body wants to be in balance and stay in balance. If something is teetering one way in the body, the body is going to do something more to make that balance come back. The first roadblock that we suffer from is hormonal imbalance.

Hormones

Hormonal imbalance can be caused from several things. First, we will look at where the hormones come from in the body. This discussion will briefly let you know about the different glands that produce the hormones that are in our body that causes our body to function properly. We will not go over this in-depth. I have more information on my website. If you think you may have any hormonal imbalance, and you may be able to tell as we go through the chapter about listening to your body and its symptoms, I strongly suggest that, if you find that you do have some hormonal symptoms, check out my website. You will be able to be further guided to possibly getting hormonal testing and or talking to your physician. On the website, you will gain an understanding of what foods may help with your hormones. Please refer to that, because the scope of this book cannot cover all the information.

There are ten glands that we have in the body that secret and give off hormones. I will just briefly name them. There is adrenal medulla, the adrenal cortex, the pancreas, the parathyroid, the thyroid, the posterior pituitary, the anterior pituitary, the pineal gland, the testes, and the ovaries. Each one of those glands secretes different hormones that help our body run smoothly. Each of these glands are important to provide the body with what it needs to be healthy.

One hormone that we are concerned about with weight loss and health is produced by the adrenals. It is cortisol. It is necessary for survival. It stimulates the stress response. But, with excessive and chronic low-grade stress, and if released too much, it will lead to fat storage around the midsection. Cortisol's function is to protect the neurons from damage and repairs the myelin sheath around the nerve. This is one of the most important hormones. It improves memory, motivation, and sleep immunity, and can contribute to PMS and menopausal symptoms.

One condition that we will talk about is hypothalamus-pituitary adrenal (HPA) axis dysfunction. HPA axis dysfunction is formally known as adrenal fatigue. We will be discussing this one a lot, because it is mainly caused by stress. It is an overproduction of cortisol and adrenaline. We have reviewed our life, investigating our foundational food groups, and we realized that we do a lot in our lives as women—a lot of stressful things. We are on the go. This influences our HPA axis or our adrenal glands. We need to consider that, when we are stressed, the limbic system—the amygdala and hippocampus; the amygdala with our emotions and the hippocampus with our memory— stimulates the hypothalamus, which is part of the HPA axis. When it stimulates the hypothalamus, it kicks in the autonomic nervous system into action, which causes us to go into fight, flight, or freeze, or rest, digest, and relax.

Of course, if we are in high stress and not relaxing, our blood flow shifts to the muscles to help us get away from the danger. When this happens, the blood is stopped from going to the gut and our food doesn't get digested too quickly because the body is working to stay away from danger. We gain weight.

The Digestive System

> *"All disease begins in the gut."*
> **– Hippocrates**

The digestive system is another reason why you're not able to lose the weight and keep it off. I want to help you understand more about why the gut is such a control system for your weight loss. Let's start with what the digestive system consists of.

I will start at the beginning: the mouth. When placing food in our mouth, we can consciously help how our food gets digested by how much we chew our food. The mouth has digestive enzymes located in the salivary glands that help to digest our food. That old saying, "Chew your food," is so true. The reason it is true is because, in the mouth, the saliva has strong digestive enzymes, that once the food particles are broken down into little tiny pieces, are released to help us chemically break it down further. Can you imagine? If you are like most of us, we take a bit of food, chew it twice, and swallow. How many of us eat our food on the go, in the car, standing at the kitchen sink, or when we are in a hurry, and we take a bite, chew three times, and swallow? Can you imagine how hard it's going to be for the stomach to digest huge parcels of food? But, if we would just chew our food, the digestive enzymes would be released, and it would be easier for the stomach to accept it.

Okay, here is another trick for you. The digestive enzymes are released as we chew. If, however, we drink water with a meal, or alcohol with the meal, the digestive enzymes will be weakened. It's okay to drink half an hour before your meal, but you want the digestive enzymes in your mouth to be able to do the best they can to help stomach.

The next part of the digestive system is the esophagus. This is the tube that connects your mouth to your stomach. It prevents food from moving up from the stomach into the esophagus by using what is called the esophageal sphincter. When we have a burning sensation or acid reflex, this is a malfunction the esophageal sphincter. This is mainly caused by eating foods that change the stomach acid's pH balance.

The next piece of the digestive tract is the stomach. The stomach is rich in an acid called hydrochloric acid. This acid helps to break down the food further. The stomach allows some nutrients to be absorbed, and it allows some liquids to be absorbed into your bloodstream. The stomach should not have any bacteria in it. The stomach needs to have a pretty clean area for us to digest our food properly. It typically has a low pH. The low pH is a defense mechanism against bacteria in the stomach. The acid is helpful in breaking down proteins and allows us to absorb nutrients and minerals. If we have low stomach acid for some reason, which would mean the stomach acid has a higher pH than normal, this could lead to bacterial growth and less functional digestive enzymes. When the enzymes in the stomach can't break down the food, we have food particles that are still not broken down, and they travel to the lower areas of the digestive tract. This is the first of the attack on the body, and it causes our bodies to suffer from inflammation.

The next part of the digestive tract is the small intestine. It is about twenty feet long. The small intestine's job is to absorb nutrients and water. It has enzymes in it that break down foods further. The enzymes that help break down the food particles further are released from the pancreas and from bile from the liver and gallbladder.

As we travel further, we come to the large intestine, or the colon. The large intestine has lots of bacteria. It is supposed to. This is where the microbiome is. The large intestine has many bacteria in it. There are over 100 trillion gut bacteria in our large intestine. Not only does the large intestine have good bacteria, it has yeast and other viruses in it. We need a good percentage of good bacteria in the gut biome. When the yeast and good bacteria are offset and out of the normal balance, we have a difficult time digesting our food.

Many studies are starting to connect weight gain to the microbiome. One study that I found particularly interesting is where the researchers took germ-free mice, biologically identical, that were in good weight and health, and mice that were raised conventionally and had forty percent higher body fat. These conventionally raised mice even ate less food than the germ-free mice. However, once the gut microbiome from the conventionally raised mice was implanted in the germ-free mice, the germ-free mice had a sixty percent increase in body fat within two weeks. The food that the mice ate was not changed nor was the activity level. The only change was the gut biome. This article was found in, Nutrition Today, "The Gut Microbiome and It's Role in Obesity" Cindy D. Davis, Ph. D.

The interesting thing about the large intestine and the gut biome is that if there is an upset in the balance of good bacteria to bad bacteria, the bad bacteria or yeast—candida—can cause particles of food to not be digested. This sets us up for the leaky gut syndrome.

The large intestine needs lots of bacteria. There are ten microbes in the gut for every cell in our body. The gut flora includes 100 trillion bacteria. We develop the microbiome from our environment. The first inoculation we have that gives us some bacteria is when we are born and come through the vaginal cavity. There are studies that show that children that do not get this first inoculation by coming through the vaginal cavity and were born with a C-section, their bodies have a hard time gaining good gut microbiota. A healthy microbiome has a good ratio of good bacteria to the bad. When we are stressed; take medication;

antibiotics; or drink diet soft drinks containing sugar-free, chemically made sweeteners, we disrupt the normal gut ratio. This sets us up for inflammation and illness.

Now, when you suffer from an illness or infection and your autonomic nervous system tries to get you better, it places your healing as its priority and turns off the rest and digest. The nervous system says, "Hey, wait a minute, I've got to take care of my person," and so it shifts all its power to getting better, not to providing digestion of the food in your stomach.

This physical stress of illness stimulates your autonomic nervous system. The system recognizes it as danger and it switches on the fight, flight, and freeze. It shifts all the blood to the muscles. The Autonomic nervous system prioritizes getting away from danger versus trying to digest your food. Weight gain occurs. Your autonomic nervous system wants the body to prevent illness from taking the host—which is you—so the gut doesn't get the blood supply and therefore it cannot operate as functionally. I want you to imagine your gut biome as a lush, beautiful garden. It is green and growing beautifully. Think about your garden without water. Okay, this is the same as not having blood flow to the digestive system. You would see your garden wilt and not be as strong and prolific, right? Same for the microbiome.

Now, also think about what happens when we take antibiotics. Think about your garden again. When you take antibiotics, your gut microbiome gets killed by the antibiotics. Antibiotics kill good bacteria and bad bacteria. They kill everything. Imagine your beautiful garden, and now you just sprayed weed killer on it. It is going to destroy all the vegetation. This is what happens to your gut microbiome when you take antibiotics. We destroy our garden. Now, I am not saying we shouldn't take antibiotics, but I do think we should be more cautious and mindful about when we take antibiotics. But more importantly, I want to you to, after taking the antibiotics, replenish the good gut bacteria by eating prebiotic foods.

The problem is that, after we take antibiotics, we leave the yeast and sugar-hungry biome behind. This offset the balance of good gut bacteria to bad. This imbalance, causes the yeast to become higher in number. I'll explain how to incorporate good gut bacteria to our system later with good foods for your digestive tract in Chapter 7, when we talk about our foods that we're going to eat.

In 1973, the first broad-spectrum antibiotic, Keflex, was produced. If you look back at the rates of obesity and how it rose, there is a strong correlation to obesity and the time of the antibiotic. What truthfully may be happening is that the sugar-hungry yeast and bacteria that is in our microbiome may be requesting sugary, processed food. The gut and brain talk to one another. If the gut wants something to feed yeast, it will signal the brain to crave sugar. Guess what happens? You can't resist that piece of cake. You're craving sugar to feed the bacteria in your microbiome.

We do know that when we take antibiotics, it is like spreading gasoline on our garden or using a weed killer on our garden. Be mindful: taking antibiotics can save lives, but we have to replenish the good gut biome after we take them.

One more thing. I would like to point your attention to the meats that we eat. If we look closely at the animals that we eat, it is important to know where they were raised and how they were raised. We know that antibiotics damage our microbiome, but what about the antibiotics that are used in our meat from factory-raised beef, chicken, pork, and lamb? The antibiotics that are given to the animals and the hormones that are given to the animals raise them to slaughtering size go directly into us when we eat that food, even if we hold off taking antibiotics ourselves. If we eat factory-raised beef that have hormones added to it and antibiotics added to it, we still pour gasoline on our beautiful garden, killing all of the good bacteria.

Other foods that we drink quite a bit of are sugar-free soft drinks. Sugar substitutes that are chemically produced are also like pouring gasoline on our garden. Duke University found that one pack of Splenda killed fifty percent of the gut microbiome. Let's learn what happens to the gut biome when it is displaced with antibiotics. The yeast survives and becomes overpopulated. That overpopulation of yeast craves sugar, processed food, and junk. Have you ever made rolls or bread from scratch? The yeast in the dough needs something to make it wake up and grow. You sprinkle some sugar on it and a little bit of warm water. The sugar feeds the yeast, it rises, and grows.

When we have a decrease in good gut bacteria, the yeast percentage grows and requests that we feed it. It wants to grow. The yeast craves sugar and processed foods. Now, it sends the message to the brain, and the brain listens. There goes your willpower. Typically, we beat ourselves up because we could not stop the craving. Our gut listened to the brain. Then you have shame, and here comes the negative self-talk. You have poor willpower, and your negative self-talk which signals the brain— "Hello." This stimulates the limbic system, and here we go again.

Other foods and medication that destroys your microbiome are nonsteroidal anti-inflammatories and drinking alcohol. While we are still in the large intestine, we might as well talk about the leaky gut that everyone is talking about. The cell wall on the large intestine is a mucous layer consisting of one single-cell-layer thick. To explain this easily, I want you to maybe think about it as tile and grout. The grout acts like the space between each cell. It is like tiles and grout connected.

When we eat processed foods, our body has a hard time breaking down the toxins. The body may not be able to break down something that has been placed in our food—possibly a preservative to extend a shelf life, as an example. Possibly, the gut microbiome has decreased blood flow to it from stress, illness, and physical trauma. This lack of blood flow to the gut causes the grout to weaken, which, in the body, would be the structures in-between the cell chain that lines the gut walls. When the good bacteria can't do its job of breaking down the processed food, the piece of food escapes through the cell wall lining of the gut and gets into the bloodstream. Normally, all the food gets digested, and the colon absorbs what is fuel for the body. When all the food is digested, it goes to the liver portal vessel leading to the liver. The liver filters the blood for detoxification prior to it circulating through the body.

If the gut leaks food particles through the cell gut lining or through the intestinal wall before the food particles are filtered by the liver, they are now in our bloodstream and cause our bloodstream to react and try to defend the body. In our bloodstream, the particles are foreign. Our blood has white blood cells, red blood cells, and interstitial fluid. The white blood cells are there to take care of invasions. They say, "Hey, what is this? This is foreign, and it is not supposed to be here." The white blood cells attack the foreign particle. It builds antibodies in our body to destroy it. The food particle is broken down into a protein molecule, and this protein molecule sometimes attaches itself to one of our organs or one of our glands. For example, if it attaches itself to the thyroid gland, it is determined to be a threat and antibodies are formed. Now that it attached to the thyroid gland, the body sees it-the thyroid gland- as that foreign particle and attacks its thyroid cells. The white blood cell says, "Hey, this is bad. I attacked you once. I need to build antibodies to protect my host from getting sick." The protein mimics the thyroid gland. The body self-destroys, and this is how an autoimmune disease starts. All because this piece of undigested food got out of the gut.

Autoimmune diseases occur in the pancreas, thyroid, the cartilage in our joints, and our nerves. The escaped particles attach and mimic those cells that are good for our body, and when it mimics the cells that are good for our body, the body still says, "Hey, wait a minute, that's something that was bad and I built antibodies against it." This is how we develop autoimmune deficiencies or illnesses: because the body attacks itself.

Traveling further, we have the liver. It is the second of the largest organs in your body. Think about the liver as a filtration system on a fish tank. It cleanses the blood of toxins. The liver breaks down the proteins into amino acids so we can use them as an energy source and nutrients to fuel our body. It also breaks down fat into the fatty acids so we can also use them. If you think about a fish tank full of water, it will be able to do a little easier job detoxifying if the tank had an adequate amount of water, right? Well, what if you were someone who did not ever drink water during the day.?

Can you imagine what a fish tank would look like with only an inch of water in the bottom of the tank? Can you imagine how difficult it would be for the filtration system to do a good job, if at all? Drink your water. Here is a little hint about water. The liver needs to filter everything in the blood before it goes to the heart to be pumped through the body. The liver detoxifies everything from the air that we breathe, the products we put on our skin, and the food that we take in. Its job is to filter through all the stuff that we give to our body. Imagine the fish tank, and let's say that one of your little vices is not drinking enough water, which was mine. Our body is seventy-five percent water. It needs water to function.

I want you to imagine the fish tank when you forget to drink your water.

The next section of the digestive tract is the gallbladder. The gallbladder is located and attached to the back of the liver. The gallbladder stores bile, which also helps break down food particles and help us with the digestions of fats.

Next is the pancreas. The pancreas sits near the small intestine and is behind the stomach. The pancreas produces hormones, insulin, and glucagon, which also helps us maintain a normal weight. The pancreas helps the body to control blood sugar levels in our system. The pancreas works overtime in this day and age secondary to the excessive sugar we are consuming.

Chakras

Another area we will look at possible reasons for weight gain and health issues is in the chakras. Our body can hold triggers of trauma in the chakras. In Eastern cultures, the chakra system is considered our center for health. The Eastern belief is that there is an energy life force that runs through our bodies. The energetic vibrational force is referred to with different names in different areas of the country. In Thailand, it is referred to as sen. In India, it is referred to as nadis. In China, it is chi. The vibrational energy has two opposite energies: yin, the more feminine, and yang, the more masculine. The chakras are a wheel of energy or light. We will talk more about this later in the book.

If the vibrational energy that is flowing through our body becomes sluggish, our chakras will have emotional, mental, and physical symptoms. Our body holds triggers in these chakras. We will discuss this in-depth later. For now, it is important to realize that when we suffer from a trauma—physically, mentally, or emotionally—we will hold the trauma in areas of our body. In the chakra system, there are seven areas, and more recently, there has been speculation of an eighth chakra. The vibrational pathways through the body will slow down or close off if we have not performed the proper healing to bring balance to our life. I experienced a blocked second chakra as I shared in Chapter 2. When I realized what trauma my body was holding on to, I was able to release the feelings and move past the blockage.

There are many reasons that our body tries to hold onto weight and tries to protect us. I can help you address these areas once we understand what and how our body is reacting to certain situations the way it does.

In this chapter, I explained how our body is affected by stress, which directly impacts our hormones. When our hormones become out of balance, our body tries to find balance by increasing or decreasing hormones in other parts of the body. I explained in depth the digestive system, which can help us understand what each organ is primarily designed to do to help us digest our foods more efficiently. As I explained, we are now aware of what may cause our digestive system to become out of balance, and we can avoid or bring balance back to our digestive system with foods we will learn about in the next chapters.

Finally, in this chapter, we learn about the Eastern philosophies of the chakra system. I want to express the importance of the chakras and the meridian system in order to be able to locate past traumas that we may be holding in our body that triggers our actions and our food choices. We are one step closer to unlocking the reason for your weight gain.

Chapter 7
What Truly Is in Your Food?

"Let food be thy medicine and medicine be thy food."
– Hippocrates

Step 4

Today, it is difficult to truly know which foods to eat. I know that some of the diets and catchy ways to lose weight may seem attractive to you. They seemed attractive to me when I tried to diet. I would try the various popular diets for about ten to fifteen days. I would count calories and grams of fat, and make sure I was getting my protein requirements, but then I would, for some reason, fail to stay on the diet. I would then punish myself for failing, eat everything in sight, and then gain ten to fifteen more pounds. I just could not figure it out. I believe what truly happened to me and other clients that suffered from the same problem is that diets just do not work. I believe that the reason we stop the diet is an emotional reason. Our body communicates back and forth from brain to gut. I believe that some triggers occur that we have buried deep inside. We will cover this more in Chapter 10.

I also believe that counting calories and trying to limit our food consumption based on nutritional data on the back of a package can be sabotaging. What I realized is all calories are not the same. Let's dive into what I mean.

When you eat a product that was prepared for you—say, a diet meal that you can buy in the frozen section at the grocery market—it has been on the shelf for, I am not sure, maybe years. There is a shelf life on this type of food to extend its longevity. When you consume this food, your body tries to digest the chemicals that preserved this food. The additives to the food to extend its shelf life make it colorful and make it taste better, and it is chemically processed, in which nutrients have been removed to use in other foods. Processed foods contain extra sugar, salt, artificial flavors, colors, chemical sweeteners, genetically modified ingredients, processed industrial oils, and unhealthy fats. Manufacturers place high amounts of sugar in the food. It makes it taste good, but it is also to increase our desire for the food. Sugar has been found to be extremely addictive.

The foods we currently eat cause inflammation in our system. Americans eat tons of sugar without realizing it. Our portion sizes increased to three times that of the 1970s. What we eat as food for fuel for our body is also causing inflammation in the body. I know how I can help people lose weight and have a successful healthy life.

Here is a quick list of the top additives to avoid in food.

Aspartame, known as 951:

This is used in diet foods to increase sweetness. It is a neurotoxin and carcinogen affecting short term memory.

High fructose corn syrup/HFCS:

Used in processed foods like bread, candy yogurts, and salad dressings.

This is the highest-used sweetener in America. It increases weight gain.

Monosodium glutamate/MSG/E621L:

Used in Chinese food, potato chips, snack foods, cookies, and seasoning.

It is a flavor enhancer and it interrupts the neuropathways to the brain that says, "I am full."

Trans fats/partially hydrogenated vegetable oils:

Increases the bad fats in our blood and contributes to heart disease and strokes.

Some examples of additives to our foods that may adverse effects to our brain and body:
- Food dyes and color additives
- Sodium sulfate
- Sodium nitrate/sodium nitrite
- BHA and BHT
- Potassium bromate
- Propyl paraben
- Aluminum additive
- Sulfur dioxide

Many on the list above are cancer-causing, neurotoxins, or endocrine-disrupting, and they will affect how our body tries to maintain its balance.

The body tries desperately to take care of you. When we eat food that our body is unfamiliar with, it will send out the troops to try and control the destruction. Unfortunately, when it is too overwhelming for the body to handle, disease sets in.

The words "refined" and "enriched" on the label means that the food has been stripped of important nutrients of the product to use in another product, then added back to the packaged food with fillers that were chemically processed. As we eat this product, it fills us up. The package states that we consumed 400 calories. The nutritional statistics are labeled on the package. The ingredient list is so long that you cannot pronounce the list of words. But we eat it and then wonder why we feel low-energy about two to three days into the diet. The truth of the matter is that the food in the package was stripped of its nutritional fiber content and refined to make it taste good. Processed foods typically are so contaminated with fillers and poor nutritional value, that we truly starve our body of nutrients. Now, one can understand the reason for feeling tired and low-energy day six into the diet. We haven't even eaten real food. Processed foods that we all reach for and cause us to feel full but do not give us any nutritional value include breakfast cereal, pizza, soda, chips, boxed rice, stovetop foods, saltine crackers, sugar, and mixes to add to your cooking. The list goes on. Processed food is typically anything that you must open from a box, bag, or can.

To avoid processed food, try to eat whole foods, fresh foods, and pasture-raised meat. If you have to eat something that you need to open, read the ingredients. I try to avoid more than six on a list, and I need to be able to identify what the foods are in the list. If there are any words you cannot pronounce, you should avoid the food.

It can be scary to think that the food we try to fuel our body with could be dangerous for us. Many of the foods that we consume have little nutritional value in them. Processed food is modified to sustain a shelf life. What our body needs for fuel are whole, unprocessed foods. A great question to ask yourself if you eat whole foods is, "If I put this in the ground (if it is a vegetable or plant product), will it grow?"

I had to laugh at myself a couple of years back. I thought I was eating so healthy, and I was compared to what I was eating like when I yo-yo-weight-dieted. Currently, I try to eat one plant-based meal per day. I would open a can of beans and make a great salad. Then, one day, I realized if tried to plant that bean from the can, would it grow? No way. When I say, Can you plant the vegetable, seed, or bean and will it sprout or grow, it should be able to, which means it is a whole food. For example, if you plant the end of a celery stalk, it will grow. Plant a bean not from a can, it will grow. One plant-based meal per day for me works for my body. Remember, every person's body is individual. What works for me, may not work for another, the trick is finding out what works best for your individual body. Not every individual body does well with a plant-based diet. It is important for you to figure out what diet works for your body. I will help you understand which diets work the best for you. As you learn to listen to your body's symptoms, you too will be able to determine if the foods, and diet you are eating is serving your body optimally. When your body is getting the correct foods for it, the symptoms will go away and your body will achieve a balance and therefore better health.

Consider how animals are raised. The environment that your protein is raised in can also affect the quality and nutritional value of your food. Factory-raised animals are in an extremely unhealthy environment for the animal. There is no room to move, they stand in their waste, and their feed is placed on their waste on the ground. One time, when I drove through California in an RV, I smelt something horrible. I got up and looked out the window, and it was a factory farm of beef cattle. They stood probably one foot apart from each other, and you couldn't even see the ground. They were so close, but what was even worse is they stood in mud, which was actually their waste. Worse yet, they were fed on the ground. The food that they consumed was all mixed with their waste. Be aware that when you eat factory-raised beef, they were fed in horrible conditions, they were given hormones to promote faster growth, and they were given a series of antibiotics.

As we discussed earlier, the gut biome is destroyed by antibiotics. When the gut biome has a decrease in the good bacteria, the bad bacteria or the sugar craving bacteria overwhelm the system and crave more sugary sweets. Thinking back to factory-raised animals. All of them. They are fed genetically modified corn to fatten them up, and they're also fed in their waste. It was a terrible sight. Try to find your meat source if you are a meat-eater from pasture-raised farmers. Chicken, beef, pork, and lamb should be purchased from a source that allows the animal to roam. The healthier the animals are, helps us to have an easier time digesting the food. We should not be asking our bodies to try to break down all the processed chemicals that come from factory-raised animals.

For our carbohydrate source, again, avoid proceeds foods. Commercially baked goods have a refined carbohydrate that is made from white flour, as we discussed previously. That flour was stripped of all its nutrients and refined. All sugars, sugary foods, and alcohol are processed. Any time you read on the label "refined" or "enriched," the food has been modified and the good nutrients have been taken out of the food and chemicals have been placed in the food to make it taste good. It fills us up faster and makes us want more of it. It is why they put a lot of sugar in commercially baked goods, dairy, sauces, and yogurt. Our body craves the sugar. Remember, sugar is addictive, and it signals the brain via the gut and the bad gut microbiome to want more.

When it comes to the fats in our diet, we want to avoid soy, corn oil, canola oil, and vegetable oil. These are just a few to avoid due to their link to accelerate heart disease. Trans fats, processed fats, and hydrogenated fats are linked to increasing infertility. Hormones need good fat and protein to work efficiently and to be able to produce a healthy body. Olive oil, avocado oil and grape seed oil (for high smoke point oil) are my go-to oils of choice.

Another area of concern that we need to be aware of that causes our body to self-destruct is what is put on our food, or how our food is raised. Genetically modified organisms (GMO), also referred to since 2018 as bioengineered food—are plants that were modified to resist insects. They also were modified to look nice and be larger. The worst GMO foods that should be avoided always are corn, soybeans, sugar beets, oilseed crops (soy, corn, canola, cottonseed oil), and corn syrup, which are made from predominantly GMO, starchy field corn.

The food itself was modified with a pesticide in it so that it kills animals and resists damage from bugs. Think about that. The food was modified to kill animals—what are we? These toxins get into our body when we eat this type of food, and our body once again tries to defend itself.

If you cannot afford to purchase organically grown vegetables, try to wash your food with a veggie wash or a do-it-yourself hydrogen peroxide wash to decontaminate the sprayed-on pesticides. It was also determined that simply washing your produce with water does not remove the chemicals. It is believed that over sixty-five percent of the produce sold in the United States was contaminated with a pesticide. A great reference to visit to find out more information about the produce you eat is ewg.org.

Europe has banned most of the products that we still eat in the United States. There are as many as 225 different types of pesticides found on our produce, and Europe doesn't allow them. A French study published in JAMA Internal Medicine found that almost 69 thousand participants that eat mostly organic foods showed twenty-five percent fewer cancers than individuals who did not eat organic. Another study performed by Harvard University in 2018 found a surprising increase in fertility issues when consuming non-organic foods.

Here is the 2019 EWG's list for the dirty dozen of most pesticide-ridden produce in order of worst to least.

1. Strawberries
2. Spinach
3. Kale
4. Nectarines
5. Apples
6. Grapes
7. Peaches
8. Cherries
9. Pears
10. Tomatoes
11. Celery
12. Potatoes

I also would like to recommend that, if you love peppers—hot peppers included—avoid these. Put them on your list of purchase only organic.

The EWG also reports a list of the clean fifteen each year. These are the cleanest vegetables and fruits, but they still contain a small amount of pesticide, so still wash them.

1. Avocados
2. Sweet corn
3. Pineapples
4. Frozen sweet peas
5. Onions

6. Papayas
7. Eggplants
8. Asparagus
9. Kiwis
10. Cabbages
11. Cauliflower
12. Cantaloupes
13. Broccoli
14. Mushrooms
15. Honeydew melons

Our bodies fight inflammation every day with exposure to toxins, foods, and stress. Inflammation is one of the leading causes of disease and illness. Here is a list of foods that cause our bodies to be stressed and get inflamed.

1. Sugar and high fructose corn syrup
2. Artificial trans fat
3. Vegetable and seed oils
4. Refined carbohydrates
5. Excessive alcohol
6. Processed meats

All the above were discussed. I like a list, so I have it ready for future references.

In order to lose your weight and help your body function more efficiently, we need to feed it with the proper nutrition. By now, you know what causes your body to be stressed and become inflamed. In the detox chapter, we will move through our pantry and home and get rid of any foods that may hurt our body. This will help us make room for the food that will help our body be stronger and rid itself of the weight that it is holding onto because of the inflammation and the survival instinct. As we have learned, we are in a constant chronic low-grade stress with our lives today. We are constantly on the go, and with this fast-passed lifestyle and the fear of missing deadlines or commitments, we have our autonomic nervous system in a state of constant stimulation to the sympathetic system. We try to survive, which shifts our blood flow away from rest and digest. We will address how to align our foundational food groups in Chapter 10. In this next section, I will educate you on good foods for your body.

From this time forward, you will think about eating only whole, unprocessed, unrefined, non-processed foods. Avoid excessive sugar and simple carbohydrate foods, such as white bread, donuts, and sugary sodas.

Every individual's body is different. What works for one person may or may not work for you. Think about foods you like and try to eat as similar to how you eat, but take into consideration that you have the choice to eat a healthy variety of the food. I typically add a shopping day to my client's program when they hire me to guide them as a health coach.

When I take the client shopping, it is interesting to see what they think is good for them and what they judge their buying decision on. Sometimes, the client looks at the price of an item, and that is how they base their purchase. I encourage you to think about what a risk you take in purchasing poor quality food versus better, less commercially treated food. Think about your body and what it is doing to it. Is it worth the risk to purchase the cheapest bag of chips with all the additives that will make you suffer from inflammation and weight gain?

I once took a client to the store for a shopping day. I said, "What do you enjoy eating?" He commented on what he enjoyed, and we headed to that section. First, he enjoyed eating green beans for a vegetable. I said, "Let's go get them." At that moment, I turned to the fresh produce and he turned to the canned vegetable aisle. Interesting, right? I know your choice would be fresh, because you now understand what happens to our food when it is processed. Remember, food should be whole, not something you open from a can, box, or bag. I encouraged the client to shop the exterior of the store, not to go in the center where all the processed food lives.

Let's find our foods that are great to eat. Just to name a few:

Proteins

Grass-fed and pasture-raised meats. This includes pork and lamb. Avoid meats that were fattened up with grain or treated with antibiotics and hormones.

Pasture-raised chicken, eggs, duck, and turkey

Wild-caught or hunted game, fish, deer, elk moose, and bison

Wild-caught, low-mercury fish

Shellfish, clams, mussels, oysters, scallops, and shrimp

Plant proteins—legumes, lentils, beans, seeds, and nuts—are a great source of soluble and insoluble fiber.

Carbohydrates consisting of grains and veggies include the following:

Grains and legumes:

Brown rice, wild rice, lentils, quinoa, millet, buckwheat (soaked), and sprouted breads

Veggies:

Stick to the clean fifteen and remember to purchase only organic in the dirty dozen. I purchase my organic veggies from a delivery service to my home. I know that all the produce is organic and comes from local farmers. I like to do this because, well, seriously, I hate to go to the grocery store. I try to purchase all my produce from farms. I also use the convenience of the pick-up-at-the-door system so many grocery stores offer. You see, when I go into the store, I spend so much more money. I guess I am a sucker for the sales or attractive marketing. I found that I save money by not going to the store. When I do go, I shop the perimeter only. Back to the veggies.

Low-glycemic-value veggies. Avoid high glycemic index veggies which cause a raise in our blood sugars levels in the bloodstream.

Eat the rainbow when it comes to veggies. Make this fun: red, purple, blue, green, yellow, orange. You can do this. Here are some great choices:

Kale, swiss chard, leafy green veggies, bitter greens, spinach, cucumbers, tomatoes, carrots, pumpkin, cabbage, cauliflower, broccoli, brussel sprouts, asparagus, avocado, turmeric, seaweed sprouts fresh herbs, and fermented veggies.

With your green, leafy vegetables, try to eat according to the season. What is available will be cheaper. Eat non-leafy cruciferous vegetables which are good for the liver. Cruciferous vegetables to eat to detox the liver are like broccoli, cauliflower, brussels sprouts, and radishes. Bitter greens are also good for the liver. These include dark leafy veggies, arugula, beet tops, kale, romaine, radicchio, watercress, Belgian endive, dandelion, broccoli rabe, and mizuna (snow pea).

Fruits

Whole fruits: Avoid juice purchased from the store. We need the fiber to slow down the sugar from going to the bloodstream so fast.

Fruits: Try to stick with berries first

Best choices are

Berries: blackberries, raspberries, blueberries, strawberries, grapefruit,

lemons, limes, fresh homemade smoothies, or vegetable juices

Nuts and Seeds

Raw, not processed, almonds; raw, soaked walnuts; pecans; pumpkin seed; brazil nuts;

Seeds; chia seeds; flaxseed; and hemp heart seeds.

Fats:

Extra virgin olive oil, avocado oil, coconut oil, grass-fed butter, olives, and nut butters (almond, cashews, and pecans). Avoid peanut butter as a fat source, because of its roasting and trans fats processing.

Sweeteners

Stevia; maple syrup; raw, local honey; and dates.

Foods to Purchase to Rebuild the Gut Microbiome:

These foods would be awesome to eat regularly, but super important to eat after taking a series of antibiotics. Raw garlic, raw jicama, raw asparagus, raw leeks, raw onions, cooked onions, raw dandelion greens, raw banana, raw Jerusalem artichoke, artichokes, leeks, chicory root, cocoa, apples, flaxseed, mushrooms (shiitake, maitake, and reishi), marine algae (spirulina), chlorella, dandelion root, and probiotics and prebiotics. Foods that feed the gut bacteria need dietary fibers that humans cannot digest. This allows the food particles to make it to the large intestine or colon, which are good for gut health. All are listed above.

Foods to Stabilize Blood Sugar

Always eat a protein, fat, and fiber together. Avoid eating carbohydrates alone. Always add a protein. You need to get your omega-3 fatty acids in to control the blood sugar. These include eggs, flaxseed, hemp seeds, oily fish, and walnuts. Foods that help with insulin resistance are alfalfa sprouts, algae, seaweed, avocado, basil, bitter melon, blueberries, broccoli, brussels sprouts, cabbage, cardamom, carob powder, cinnamon cucumber, garlic ginger, greens, Jerusalem artichoke, onion, and turmeric. Can you see how the lists overlap?

Hormonal healthy choice of food are all listed above. The important factor to remember for eating to improve your hormones is to avoid processed foods and refined foods, high sugar foods, and stress.

Now you have the actual foods you should avoid and the ones to gravitate toward. There are a wide variety of foods. I gave you only a few that I tend to go to. I briefly shared only some of the foods that will be healthy and set you on a path to better health and weight loss. It is important to remember that each body will be truly unique to what it needs to perform optimally. That is why I only placed a few food items in this chapter. For example, my body does well with meat-based protein. However, I had a client that, after we researched his body's individual needs, was more successful with his weight loss by avoiding meat.

This client was constantly suffering from achiness and feelings of fatigue. He initially was eating meat daily. I noticed that, in his daily food journal that he sent me each week for his weekly recap, on the days he would eat a plant-based diet, he would report feeling happier, lighter, and less heavy. I encouraged him to adjust his food plan to having one or two days with meat protein. He felt better and his weight came off easily. Of course, this was what his body required to lose his weight and find a balance of health. He did extremely well with my program. He mainly had three goals he wanted to achieve: weight loss, decreasing his pain, and achieving a good night's sleep. He achieved all three. Once you listen to your body and feed it the appropriate food, you also on your path to losing weight and gaining energy.

Top Toxins to Avoid (from Food Matters TV)

Environmental Toxins
- Pesticides, Fungicides & Herbicides (carcinogenic)
- Fluoride (neurotoxin)
- Mercury & Lead (neurotoxin and immunosuppressant)
- EMF & EMR—Electromagnetic Frequencies and Radiation (possibly carcinogenic)
- Phthalates (hormone disruptor)

Found In: non-organic produce, tap water, amalgam fillings, mobiles, scented candles and air fresheners.

Household
- Volatile Organic Compounds (respiratory issues)
- Petroleum Solvents (damages airways)
- Formaldehyde (carcinogen)
- Butyl Cellosolve (organ damage)
- Phthalates (hormone disrupter)
- Nonylphenol
- Ethoxylates (hormone disruptor)

Found In: Non-natural cleaning products, laundry detergents and dishwasher powders.

My favorite cleaner and household products that I use are from H20@home. The cleaning supplies are not only non-toxic, but also, they use water and the fibers of the cleaning cloths to sanitize the household. I highly encourage you to try these products out. It is the fibers in the cloth that lifts the dirt, not harmful chemicals or toxins.

http://www.myh2oathome.com/krisg

Beauty and Personal Hygiene
- Parabens (hormone disruptor)
- Sodium Lauryl Sulfate (toxicity)
- Dioxin (toxic byproduct of bleach)
- PEG Compounds (increases absorption toxins)
- Phthalates & Synthetic Fragrances (hormone disruptor)

Found In: Non-organic cosmetics, soaps, perfumes, tampons, deodorants, sanitary pads & lotions.

My favorite cleaning facial clothes again are from H20@home. The cloth takes off every single bit of mascara without any soap or oil—truly amazing.

http://www.myh2oathome.com/krisg

Packaging
- Bisphenol A (BPA) (lowers fertility)
- BPS (close to BPA) (disrupts hormones)
- Polystyrene (leaches styrene)
- Polyvinyl Chloride (breaks down into toxic chloride)
- Phthalates (hormone disruptor)
- Dioxin (carcinogen and endocrine disruptor)

Found In: plastic bottles, food storage containers & cling wrap.

I use mason jars and glass containers to hold my food prep items, never plastic.

Chapter 8
Your Body Is Calling. Are You Listening?

"Turn your wounds into wisdom"
– Oprah Winfrey

Step 5

The body is so amazing. I know I keep saying this, but it is so true. It is our ego that destroys our body. Do you remember a time in your life where you might have fallen? I am sure it hurt you, but what did you do when it happened? Most people try to walk it off: brush it out of their mind, like it didn't happen, avoid feeling the pain, and mentally check out of the fall.

I cannot tell you how many times clients came to me and said their symptoms just started one day out of the blue. I typically asked them if they fell in the past. Everyone says no initially, because we want to just get moving and avoid the embarrassment. But what typically happens is, they will come back and say, "Hey, you know, I did have a nasty skiing fall about six months ago." The reason this is important is because we were taught at a young age that we need to push through the pain. My father's favorite saying when I would fall down was, "Come over here and I will pick you up," and then he would say, "Stop crying."

We stopped listening to our bodies a long time ago, and now we can't even feel them when they fail. How many times do you wait to go to the bathroom? You just push away the feeling until it is so bad you can't stand it. Let me tell you to stop doing that. You are training your bladder to become incontinent in the future.

What I am trying to impress upon you is we need to listen to our body and listen to our gut feelings. We need to become more mindful of what is happening to us. I believe that most people walk around feeling horrible. They are tired, stiff, short of breath, and lacking energy, and they don't even realize it until the symptoms turn into a disease or chronic illness.

Or, better yet, they do change what they eat and stop poisoning their bodies with the chemicals in processed foods, and they suddenly feel great and, at that time, realize how terrible they felt. Listen to your body.

The major and most telling symptom that our body has to show us that there is an imbalance is not being able to sleep. When we do not get enough sleep, this leads to weight gain and poor health.

The most probable reasons for not being able to sleep are excessive cortisol, hormonal imbalances, anxiety, and/or stress.

Sleep deprivation impacts the body system significantly. When we are in a constant state of stress, our adrenals work overtime and pump out increasing amounts of cortisol. In our fast-paced world, this causes a decrease in the production of melatonin. We need melatonin in our body for our body to sleep. Melatonin is released normally from our body when the sun goes down and it is dark. The pineal gland is responsible for the release of melatonin. When we have high cortisol levels, the melatonin production in our body is decreased. Not only does poor sleep make for a rough day the next day, it causes us to hold onto weight and have decreased ability to think clearly. When we have poor sleep, this increases our appetite, blood pressure, and heart rate. It will also cause us to feel depressed and sluggish.

Without sleep, our immune system becomes weakened, and we also make poorer food choices and, therefore, gain weight. Good sleep, on the other hand, increases the proper functioning of the prefrontal cortex, allowing for better communication between the prefrontal cortex and the limbic system. Sleep is important for regulating the serotonin level in our body (the neurotransmitter that improves our mood, willpower, and drive). A good night's sleep also increases the release of the neurotransmitter norepinephrine (our thinking, focusing, and calming neurotransmitter), which is important for being able to appropriately respond to stress. Sleep also supports healthy habits and affects the brain's reward circuitry. A bad night's sleep makes the brain respond to short term rewards like, "I want a donut now," versus long term rewards like weight loss.

Sleep helps relieve pain and helps our body and brain detox from the day's activities. When you cannot sleep, one or more of the following hormones may be off. Here are some examples of the body's symptoms and how it is trying to tell you there is something wrong.

High Cortisol Symptoms in Your Body

Let's start with high cortisol. It occurs with high levels of stress, and our society demands a high, chronic level of stress on us daily. When your body has high cortisol levels, it will respond by showing you some of these symptoms: feeling "tired, yet wired" at night, difficulty falling asleep and staying asleep, gaining weight around your belly, and pinkish-purple stretch marks on your belly thighs or back. Increased cortisol levels cause you to have increased sugar cravings, feel anxious and nervous, and feel forgetful at times. Your blood pressure may be high, you may experience indigestion or acid reflux, and you may retain water and feel puffy, especially in your hands and ankles. Your skin may show signs of high cortisol with dryness and acne. I suffered from rosacea throughout my late twenties into my mid-thirties, even though my doctor told me it was just my age. I never had my hormones checked until I was so exhausted I just wanted to lie down wherever I was.

Weight gain pattern for high cortisol is a muffin top.

Extreme fatigue is another symptom your body will tell you.

I once was watching my children play on the big toy we had in the back yard. I was so tired, I thought to myself, "How comfortable the pea gravel looked." I laid down and fell asleep. Don't be like me and most of the women I know. Listen to your body—it will tell you when there is something going on. If you feel that you are extremely fatigued like I was, try to find a functional MD to help you get to the root of the problem and test your hormones.

Hypothalamus-Pituitary Adrenal Axis Dysfunction Symptoms

Symptoms of Hypothalamus-pituitary Adrenal Axis (HPA axis). The HPA is neuroendocrine system that allows our body to perceive and manage stress. It is a complex set of information and feedback loops for our body when we experience a stressful situation. It consists of three areas in the brain: the hypothalamus, the pituitary, and the adrenals. I discussed this earlier when we talked about what stress does to our body. This system controls the reaction to stress, and in the process, it regulates many body processes, such as digestion, mood, emotions, and energy usage.

Symptoms of HPA axis malfunction include depression, brain fog, anxiety, sleeping problems, blood pressure issues, thyroid dysfunction, immune system compromises, poor blood sugar control, and increased abdominal fat. Other symptoms include feeling fatigued in the morning and mid-afternoon, slow winding down, wound healing is decreased or slow, salt cravings, dizziness when moving from sitting to standing, low sex drive, and poor muscle tone.

Low Cortisol Symptoms

Symptoms of low cortisol levels, which can occur from being in excessive stress and having high cortisol levels for extended periods of time, include salt cravings, low blood pressure, and dizziness when standing up. Further symptoms may include feelings of being tired in the morning and not wanting to get out of bed-still tired in the morning, or you may have a hard time staying asleep at night. Emotionally, you may cry for no reason or feel like life is difficult and always challenging you. You may feel depressed, and you may be hyper-reactive to stressful situations, like blowing things up in your mind over minor situations.

Estrogen Dominance Symptoms

Our body is amazing at showing us estrogen imbalances. What typically causes the estrogen dominance are high cortisol levels, low progesterone, xenoestrogens (manmade chemicals that mimic estrogen), excessive body fat, and excessive consumption of alcohol.

The symptoms it may reveal to us for estrogen dominance include heavy menstrual bleeding, breast tenderness, PMS, fibroids, menstrual migraine headaches, moodiness, endometriosis, crankiness for no reason, and weeping for no reason. You also may have mid-cycle ovulation pain. Weight gain is the same for low progesterone. If you have high estrogen, then this forces you to have low progesterone. Weight is typically in the buttocks. You may have a muffin top or more weight on your hips and thighs.

Low Estrogen Symptoms

Low estrogen, on the other hand, will show up with a decrease in your sex drive, light or no periods at all, vaginal dryness, and painful sex. You may suffer from hot flashes, joint pain, dry and aging skin, and depression.

Low Progesterone Symptoms

Body symptoms of low progesterone—I hope you see a pattern here—which is affected and decreases with the presence of high cortisol, caused by too much stress. With low progesterone, you may have a difficult time getting pregnant and staying pregnant. You may have break through bleeding mid-way in your cycle, PMS, irregular periods, bloating in the tummy, and swollen and painful breasts. Headaches near your period are common. Your body may develop fibroids on your uterus or ovaries, endometriosis, and breast cysts. Sometimes, you may even have restless legs at night, where your legs twitch. Weight gain is typically noticed on the buttocks, thighs, and hips, giving you the classic pear-shaped figure.

Moving along.

High Testosterone Symptoms

When the body has high testosterone levels, it will show you by facial acne; oily skin and hair; male-pattern baldness; hair growth on your chin, upper lip, breasts, and stomach; breast shrinkage or sagging; and dark discoloration under armpits. You may suffer from ovarian cysts or polycystic ovarian syndrome (PCOS). You may experience pain in the middle of your menstrual cycle and a longer than twenty-eight-day menstrual cycle—it maybe going to thirty-five-day cycles. Are you constantly hungry? The weight gain pattern for low testosterone is gaining weight on the back or "bra fat," around the gut, the apple shape, or the famous beer belly.

Low Testosterone Symptoms

Low testosterone body symptoms include low sex drive, painful sex, low self-confidence, decreased muscle mass, muscle weakness, lack of motivation, difficulty with concentration, low drive, bone loss or osteoporosis, sagging skin, back of arm flap, and, sadly, hair loss. Weight gain is soft fat around the belly.

Underactive Thyroid Gland Symptoms

Symptoms of an underactive thyroid gland include hair loss on your scalp, dry and brittle nails, loss of hair on your eyebrow or eyelashes, thinning hair, muscle and/or joint pain, and cold and/or tingling in your hands and feet. Do you experience hives? When you look at your tongue, there may be indents on the sides. Do you have a large thyroid gland? Finally, are you always tired?

Insulin Resistance Symptoms

The body can also give you signs that can indicate possible insulin resistance, or high blood sugar level problems: craving sweets and carbohydrates, always feeling hungry, forgetfulness, feeling tired after a meal or lightheaded when you haven't eaten, eating relieves fatigue, need to urinate frequently, and vision changes. There may be discolored patches of skin under your armpits, on back of your neck, and/or on your groin. When you are hungry, do you suffer from "hangry" symptoms? Do you become cranky and want to eat right now? Weight gain shows up with your waist girth being larger than your hip girth. Sometimes, with poor blood sugar levels, women can slowly develop PCOS and become leptin resistant.

Leptin is a hormone. It is produced in our fat cells, and it is our bodies communication hormone to the brain that says we have enough energy stored in our fat cells to slow down eating. It tells the brain, "Hey, I am full now." This causes us to stop eating. With leptin resistance, our brain doesn't get the signal to stop eating. We then overeat. Overweight people have high levels of leptin and are leptin resistant. Their brain isn't getting the signal to stop. When our body has too low blood sugar levels, it can show up as jitteriness, anxiety, unfocused thinking, impatient and angry moments, and a strong desire to have sugar to bring you back up.

Gut Imbalances and Symptoms

Let's look at some of the symptoms the body will show us if we have gut issues. The four most common gut issues are leaky gut, small intestine bacterial overgrowth (SIBO), yeast overgrowth, and fatty liver disease. All these diseases cause inflammations in the gut. The body will give the following symptoms for these conditions: gas, bloating, diarrhea or constipation, abdominal cramping and pain, chronic fatigue, low energy, depression, and anxiety. If you have too much yeast—namely, candida albicans—and a high microbe count of bad gut bacteria in your gut—possibly from antibiotics—you may have mucous-y bowel movements, frequent yeast infections, eczema, itchy ears, and a white coating on your tongue. One interesting fact: If you do suffer from leaky gut or SIBO, you will have a difficult time eating foods that have a high histamine release in them. For example, if you find yourself itching, flushing, suffering from a headache, wheezing and sneezing after eating fermented, cured, or soured foods like yogurt, lunch meats, pickles, sour cream, aged cheese, citrus, alcoholic beverages, nuts and walnuts, tomatoes, smoked fish, and dairy, this may be a sign that your body cannot tolerate these foods and you could have gut issues.

Liver Imbalance and Symptoms

When your liver is suffering from processing all the toxins and eating too many simple carbohydrates, you may notice breakouts of acne on your forehead and dark circles and puffiness under the eyes. Your skin may have a yellow cast to it as well as the whites of your eyes.

Fascial Symptoms That May Be Indicative of an Imbalance in the Body

Some fun facts to share: If the stomach is irritated, it will show facial breakouts on the corners of the mouth, upper lip, lower check, and nose.

Lungs and heart issues may show breakouts on the checks and bridge of the nose. Kidney issues show breakouts on the temples, brow lines, corners of the eyes, and under the eyes. Hormonal imbalance breakouts will show up on the jawline, mainly caused from stress.

Can you now begin to see why stress is the underlying factor to weight gain and inflammation in the body? With hormonal imbalances, there is a greater risk of getting an autoimmune disease, where the body attacks itself. Some examples of an autoimmune disease are rheumatoid arthritis, Sjögren's syndrome, Hashimoto's thyroiditis, Graves' disease, lupus, chronic fatigue syndrome, and fibromyalgia. These illnesses were researched, and there was a link found that it can be possibly due to high estrogen levels.

Listen to your body. It will share with you some valuable information that will not only help you lose that weight but also help you prevent an illness from turning into a chronic disease. It is important that we watch out for signs and symptoms that could help us get on top of balancing our hormones.

Let's peek at how Eastern Cultures listen to their bodies.

Eastern Philosophies and Symptomology

Another way your body may tell you that something is wrong is to look at it through the Eastern philosophy methods of health and wellness. If we look at chakras, we can be informed of areas that may be restricted.

The restrictions will show up with emotions, repeated thoughts, and actions, and body alignments that we tend to stay stuck in. The word "chakra" comes from the Sanskrit word for "wheel of light." Chakras are energy centers in our body that receive energy from the earth. There originally was thought to be seven chakras of the body, but currently there is mention of an eighth chakra. We will discuss the first seven only.

Each chakra is associated with an emotional, psychological, and physical issue and an area of the body. The chakras form a link between our vibrational energy anatomy to our physical anatomy of nerves, hormones, and emotions. When there is a trauma that we suffer, whether it is physical, emotional, or mental, the chakras will absorb the energy and become sluggish or stuck at its level that corresponds to that chakra level. The energy will fail to move, and the body may suffer from emotional pain or mental/physical symptoms in that chakra.

When chakras are in balance, there is a free flow of energy to and from the body. It comes up through the earth, and this is a more female or a "drawing in" force. It is more feminine in nature. There is another flow of energy from above that goes down through the body, and this is more masculine. The different chakras operate at different vibrational frequencies. When all the chakras are in alignment, they operate and flow with the universal energy. There is a sense of balance. The body interacts with and receives energy from universal energy, energy from nature, and other people's energies. If something causes a trauma to the individual, one or many of the chakras may become blocked. There is a loss of flow, and it sets the body up for illness or emotional blockages.

Each chakra is associated with a gland in the endocrine system. The heathy body has an equal amount of opposite energies. The energy can be either a male (yang) and or a feminine (yin) one. When discussing the emotional and physical attributes of the chakras, realize that there is a balance. If the chakra is out of balance, the behavior of the person can swing to the extremes.

The Root Chakra Symptoms

The root chakra is located at the bottom of our spine and governs the feet, knees, legs, and pelvic region. It is linked to the adrenal gland.

The color of root chakra is red. When in balance, the person feels grounded, stable, and secure. When it is less active, the individual may feel fearful/nervous and they do not feel like they belong to their tribe. An overactive root chakra can show up in the individual as greediness and materialistic. It is mainly responsible for our survival process and basic needs. It relates to our childhood experiences. A good childhood leads to faster transcendence and a balanced first chakra, while an unpleasant and unsafe childhood often leads to anxiety, depression, and trauma, which indicate the blockage in root chakra. Emotionally, this chakra allows us to feel safe and have a sense of belonging to a tribe or family. It helps us rate where we stand in our tribe, if we feel safe in our tribe, and if we feel safe in the world. Its attributes are self-confidence, peacefulness, vitality, focus, and courage. It provides us with the ability to trust or not trust. It allows us to find our independence. Some physical symptoms that may show up if there is a loss of flow in this chakra include chronic spinal pain, back pain, sciatica, rectal tumors, chronic fatigue, fibromyalgia, arthritis, and autoimmune diseases.

The Sacral Chakra Symptoms

The sacral chakra is mainly responsible for sexual activities and attraction. The gland associated with is the testes in men and ovaries in women. The color is orange. It is all about feeling and sexuality. When in balance, the individual is open to intimacy and lives passionately and happily. When it is out of flow, the individual appears stiff, unemotional, and not interested in other people. If the chakra is overactive, the individual may be overemotional and can become emotionally attached to people too quickly. It balances our desires in the outer world with our drives we try to achieve in the form of sex, power, money, and our relationships. It allows us to be dependent or co-dependent. It is where we learn to set boundaries and define our assertiveness or lack of assertiveness. It helps us have the capability to attach to, or lack of interaction and attraction with opposite sex.

The attributes of the sacral chakra are creativity, self-worth, wisdom, energy, and self-expression. This chakra regulates the reproductive organs, kidneys, lower intestines, hips, bladder, and gallbladder. The energetic function of the second chakra is to maintain emotional balance. Some emotional issues one suffers from because of this chakra can be fear of abandonment, fear of financial security, and fear of social status. Physical problems can be seen in the form of ob-gyn problems: infertility, fibroids, cysts, pain in the pelvis, or lower back pain. It can also show up as urinary problems and appendicitis. Remember my story? My father died when I was young, I emotionally felt abandoned, I therefore had a blockage in this chakra and was not able to conceive.

The Solar Plexus Chakra Symptoms

Solar plexus chakra: This chakra is the navel chakra. It is responsible for willpower, knowledge, self-esteem, self-confidence, self-worth, and self-respect. Solar plexus chakra governs the pancreas gland. The color of solar plexus chakra is yellow. When in balance, the individual has a high self-esteem and feels in control. When underactive, the person may feel passive, indecisive, and timid. When overactive, the individual may be dominating and aggressive. Some of the attributes of the solar plexus include power, self-confidence, strength, reason, and sense of humor. Physically, the solar plexus chakra controls the stomach, upper intestines, pancreas, and lower back muscles. On an energetic level, its function is to optimize personal power and life purpose. Areas that show up emotionally when out of balance in this chakra show up with feelings of inferiority, irresponsibility, or taking on too much responsibility. The person can be aggressive or act defensive, competitive or noncompetitive, or have too many boundaries. The person may feel overly responsible.

The Heart Chakra Symptoms

Heart chakra: It is essentially responsible for love and communication. It is connected to thymus gland. The color is green. The main attributes of this chakra are love: self-love, love for others, compassion, peace, and happiness. When balanced, the person is compassionate and friendly. Your relationships are good. When underactive, the individual is cold and distant. When overactive, the individual may suffocate people with clinginess and selfish reasoning. The body regions it is associated with are the heart, the lungs, the upper back, the shoulders, the arms, the chest, the breasts, and the immune and circulatory systems. The function of the heart chakra is unconditional love. Physical symptoms of an unbalanced heart chakra can include chest pain, heart problems, asthma, allergies, lung cancer, breast cancer, and upper back and shoulder pain.

The Throat Chakra Symptoms

Throat chakra: This chakra is responsible for speech and expression. Be true to yourself. Throat chakra governs the action of thyroid gland and the respiratory system. The color for this chakra is blue. The physical body parts include the thyroid, trachea, throat, mouth, jaw, and teeth. When balanced, the individual has great self-expression and creativity. When underactive, the person is introverted and shy. They may not speak their feelings. When overactive, the person may talk too much and be domineering. Physical symptoms include bronchitis, hoarseness, chronic sore throats, mouth ulcers, jaw pain, cervical spine pain, swollen glands in the neck, and thyroid issues.

The Third Eye Chakra Symptoms

The third eye chakra: This chakra is responsible for psychic and intuitive abilities. It allows us to know ourself-mentally, emotionally and spiritually. It is associated with the pituitary gland, pineal gland, and the autonomic nervous system. The color is indigo. It is our intuition and brings psychic clarity, inner knowledge, and vision. On a physical level, the third eye manages the brain, mental processes, eyes, sinuses, nose, and ears. When in balance, the individual is intuitive. When underactive, the individual is dependent on others, may have rigid thinking, or is easily confused. When overactive, this chakra causes the person to live in a fantasy world. Physical symptoms include brain tumors, neurological disturbances, blindness, deafness, dizziness, ringing in the ears, Parkinson's disease, learning disabilities, and seizures.

The Crown Chakra Symptoms

The crown chakra is responsible for spiritual growth. It is the center for thought, truth, enlightenment, and being one with the world. This chakra regulates the pineal gland and is associated with the central nervous system. It governs the top of the spinal cord, pain centers, the spinal nerves, and brain stem. It can involve any organ system. The color of this chakra is violet. When in balance, one will be non-judgmental and at one with the world. If underactive, they are at a loss to their spirituality. If overactive, the individual may be rigid in their thinking and could be ignoring bodily needs. Physical symptoms include serious illnesses, such as multiple sclerosis, amyotrophic lateral sclerosis (ALS), multisystem failure, or any life-threatening illness or accident that serves as a wake-up call.

I would like to share a client that did well with my program. She was a mid-thirty-year-old woman that was suffering from extra weight, neck pain, and difficulty with her speech. She expressed a desire to want to lose some extra mid-thirty weight gain, but also wanted to feel more relaxed with her life. As I went through her foundational food groups, I noticed that she repeatedly had a difficult time expressing her desires and needs to others. She would continually opt to allow the other person, whether it was a co-worker, her children, or her mate, to voice their opinions and overrule hers. She suffered from chronic throat difficulties.

She, at one time, lost her voice for three years and was never able to communicate with more than a whisper.

When we addressed some of her hidden triggers in her chakras, freed some of the blockages in her meridian system, and addressed her accessory breathing—which was contributing to stress and stimulation of the fight or flight autonomic nervous system—she had less pain and anxiety. As the anxiety and pain decreased, her body relaxed, mainly by adjusting her breathing to stimulate the rest and relax autonomic nervous system state. She lost weight with only minor adjustment to her food. I evaluated her food diary and encouraged her to look at the days when she felt anxious, felt increased pain, and lost stamina. She realized those were the days she was eating more processed foods, which caused her inflammation. Shortly after that, her weight dropped off, she regained her voice, and she finally felt more in control of her life.

It is truly exciting to realize that by listening to your body and adjusting minor things in our lives, our body will drop the weight and reach a balanced equilibrium state. I shared in-depth what different parts of the body may be telling you. I would like to encourage you to write down how you feel emotionally, physically, and mentally each evening and morning on your food diary sheet. I know this may seem daunting, but it isn't. You can do it on an app on your phone or on a note pad. It may look like this (before you start eating better):

Morning: Woke up feeling slightly tired and sad,

Breakfast was eggs, bacon, potatoes, and toast. Noticed a headache and loose stools in the afternoon.

Wasn't hungry until lunch.

Lunch: I enjoyed a Caesar salad—no extra protein.

I was hungry in two hours and wanted a nap.

At three, I had to have a candy bar because I was so tired and hungry. Decided to have a vanilla latte.

So hungry on the way home I stopped at a fast food drive in. Ordered a diet Coke and fries to hold me over.

Wanted a glass of wine to cook dinner.

Needed something quick, so I ate boxed mac and cheese....

You get the idea. It isn't about counting calories or nutrients. It is about looking at what you eat. Now that you know what different foods do to your system, you will begin to realize that maybe you also feel mentally, emotionally, and physically challenged with your choices. This will help you limit those choices to better choices to avoid symptoms of pain, burping, sluggishness, et cetera.

Chapter 9
It's Time to Detox Your Life

"The first step in crafting a life you want is getting rid of everything you don't."

– Joshua Becker

Step 6

Now, you learned that it is more than food that causes our weight gain and our body to show signs of wear and tear. We noticed that it is a little harder to get out of a chair or walk up a hill. We are a little shorter in breath and patience. We learned that our body requires both foundational foods that feed our spirit and soul and food we eat by mouth that feeds our biological cells. Now, it is time to throw out the foods that no longer serve us and the foods that harm us and cause our decline in peace and calmness that is ours to have. We deserve the happiness that we were born into this world to have. It as Gabrielle Bernstein says: "Happiness is our birth right." Let's get that feeling back now. It is time to detox.

In this chapter, we will look at our foundational food groups first, and then our food we eat second. I will break it down into sections. At the end of the book, you will have a resource of where you can find lists of toxic foods, skin care products, and home items. You can also visit my website, www.SueSealWellness.com.

First, we will detox your words.

"Sticks and stones may break your bones, but words will never hurt you." This is furthest from the truth. It is like saying there is an Easter bunny that jumps around our house and leaves candy. Our words are one of the most impactful aspects of our lives. Here is what happens with words, and I am talking about your words to yourself. Remember when we talked about how the brain tries to make signals that it is familiar with? It tries to have synaptic transmissions that reach a destination. When the brain can attach a pathway to a destination it feels good, it has done its job, so to speak. Well, when you say a word—let's just say you say, "I am worthless"—the brain searches for a signal to the limbic system that will be able to make its connection. Once it is there, it can allow that system to do its job. In the case of telling yourself you are worthless; a series of reactions occur. Your limbic system talks to the hippocampus, which talks to the hypothalamus, which sends messages to the adrenals. Cortisol is released, and we are ready to fight the tiger. We no long are at rest and digest, so, once again, we cause weight to be held onto. Great, huh? Now, let us look at how the energy of the universe or the what you give you will receive.

"We are shaped by our thoughts; we become what we think. When the mind is pure, joy follows like a shadow that never leaves."
– Buddha

What this does to our energy is it creates a vibration that surrounds us and attracts similar vibrational frequencies to come our way. We now have sent out to the universe to believe that we are worthless. That vibrational frequency will now be like one in our body. All organs have vibrational frequencies. Let's say it is on the same frequency as the liver (hypothetically—this is just an example). Now, you have set the course of illness. Let's look at how the body and its energy also gathers this information. Shame and guilt will hit the spleen and stomach. This will cause stagnation in this system, and with that, we will develop the so-called "clogged pipes." With this stagnation comes inflammation, and inflammation causes illness.

One of the ways I like to look at words is as from a great book, *The Four Agreements: A Practical Guide to Personal Freedom* by Don Miguel Ruiz. He describes in his book how words are powerful and that they should be used as such. The words you use to yourself or to others should be used great care. In the book, he describes use "impeccable words," meaning what you say needs to be thought of with integrity and intention.

Talking negatively to yourself is destructive. It not only causes your body to stimulate the fight or flight, but it also causes the universe to listen to what you say. Lastly, words lead to emotional blockages in your energetic flow. Be mindful about what you say to yourself. For example, "This is hard." Well, you turned on the signal in your brain, the universe, and the bodies vibrational energy system. It will be hard now.

"A man is but the product of his thoughts.
What he thinks, he becomes"
—Mahatma Gandhi

The Home We Live In

What we surround ourselves with is what we will manifest. Let's walk through your home. First, let me share a story of when I was twenty-one. Remember, I didn't stop in my life to breath. I just kept going. Well, I wanted to learn more about why things kept happening to me. I wondered why good things would happen and then bad things would happen. For some reason, I gravitated to a Feng Shui book. I learned that what you surrounded yourself with could cause energy to change based on what and how your home was. In a nutshell, the front door is the mouth of your home. It is where everything feeds your house. Your windows are its eyes and the walls are its ears. Energy will flow through your home just like it does through the universe and through the body.

With that said, do you trip on dirty clothes? Is there clutter lying around? The clutter in your home will do two things: To our body mind, it will cause a system to be set off in the brain. Maybe it is frustration—"Where are my keys?" Now comes the frantic looking: under the piles of clothes, in the drawers, under the bed—it goes on. Then comes the angry talk—maybe you yell at the dog, who is just following you around as you rush madly and franticly through the house. Now comes the awesome words you tell yourself. "If I was more organized!" or "if I kept this house picked up better, I would not have this problem!" or maybe, "If I just freaking had time to pick this house up, this wouldn't happen to me!!" Well, the brain takes its little trip again, and bam. Injection of stress hormone once again. The weight is going to just stay right where it is.

Detox your pantry. Take the list from the previous chapter and look at your labels. If there is anything that you cannot pronounce or is longer than six ingredients on the container, make the choice to have a healthier body. Help your body lose the weight by avoiding the toxic chemicals that are in that food. Remember, our body cannot digest the processed food. It causes inflammation in our gut, in our brain, and in our body. Let me ask you this: If you had a favorite pet, would you feed it rat poison? Then why do you eat stuff that you now know makes you hold weight, become inflamed, and suffer from illness.

You see how all this works? It is a loop, and the loop is the same. Let's declutter the house using one of my favorite books, *The Life Changing Magic of Tidying Up: The Japanese Art of Decluttering and Organizing* by Marie Kondo. I witnessed it change a woman from being fearful and paranoid to successful and feeling blessed with her life. Another book I just love is *The Happy Home: Your Guide to Creating a Happy, Healthy, Wealthy Life* by Patricia Lohan.

You will be amazed at how nice it is to come into your house, place your purse in the same spot, breathe in the energy from your house, and see it welcome you. It does affect how you feel and how your health will be.

What about the chemicals we place on our bodies. This can be body products, perfume, cleaning supplies, and laundry soap. I will give you a list at the end of this chapter, and I think it will be helpful. Don't freak out about what to do. Pick one room—maybe the laundry room—and check out what you use. Change, maybe first, the fabric softener. I use wool balls, and they work amazing. But I can see you right now. Stop freaking out. Take baby steps. It took me over a year to get my home less toxic. I slowly changed my makeup and my hair products only as I needed to purchase new ones. My favorite facial and home cleaning product is called H20 at Home. Please see the back of the book to find out how to purchase this awesome product. I love how I can just use water to clean my make up off and clean my house without chemicals. Here is where I get mine: https://www.myh2oathome.com/krisg.

Don't go broke trying to change everything at once but do realize that your liver will love you for it. Remember, the liver must break down everything that we put on our skin or come in contact with. If it is working so hard to break down the toxins on our skin or chemicals that we are exposed to, how will it be able to breakdown our food and filter what it needs to in order to keep our body processing clean? With our environment, the air pollution, the additive to our foods, and the BPA pollutants, our liver is already working overtime. It is trying to filter the food, alcohol, and processed food. If it is working too hard, it will not be able to get rid of all the toxins and be able to balance all the estrogen and hormones, which is part of its job. Look at the list at the end of this chapter and realize that it is baby steps. Just having the knowledge of what your body must do will helps you make better choices.

Detox the people in our lives that are not giving you love and energy. It is true: What your surround yourself with, you become more like. I love this quote. It is in my kitchen and I try to read it as often as I need.

"People are often unreasonable and self-centered…
Forgive them anyway.
If you are kind, people may accuse you of ulterior motives…
Be kind anyway.
If you are honest, people may cheat you… Be honest anyway.
If you find happiness, people may be jealous… Be happy anyway.
The good you do today may be forgotten tomorrow…
Do good anyway.
Give the world the best you have, and it may never be enough…
Give your best anyway.

For in the end, it is between you and God.
It never was between you and them anyway."
– **Mother Teresa**

I believe that, as The Four Agreements book states, we shouldn't take things personally. People in our lives are sometimes right in the same place that we are, and sometimes they are not. Everyone has the right to be on their own journey. They may be hurtful to you at some part of your life. They may expect you to make them happy. It isn't your job to do this. Your job is to make your life happy. We cannot help other people find happiness, just as we cannot expect others to bring us our happiness. When a person in your life is trying to make you do something that you don't want to—whether they use tears or angry voices—it is up to you to look out for yourself and remove yourself from their presence. The demand of others on us, can be harmful to our health and is harmful to our bodies. We cannot be responsible for anyone but ourselves.

There were many people in my life that took advantage of my disease to please. They asked me to have parties for them, or they said, "Please, you do this so well, can't you do it for me also?" Of course, I am guilty of wanting to please everyone. Now, I learned that some people will take advantage of that kindness. Detox the people that can't accept you for what you are or what you are willing to give. Your true friends love you for who you are and they accept "no" with grace. People that push when you have said no, or, worse yet, give tears or use harsh words to force you to accommodate them—they are not your true friends. Walk away.

Now, we need to unplug our Wi-Fi. There are studies that support that the EMC that the computers and phones and TV limit causes our body inflammation and a physical stress. Place a limit on how much you do. If you need to wear blue block glasses, get them. Please do not plug your phone in next to your bed. We haven't had phones long enough to know if they can cause significant damage to our bodies. Take a page from the olden days and stop electronic social media at 9:00 p.m. The brain wants to feel okay going to bed. The next time you look at Facebook or Snapchat before going to bed, you just sent your brain a worry, your brain is trying to relax, don't stir up your amygdala now.

The tools you use to cook with may also be a concern. The best pans to use are carbon steel, cast iron, or ceramic. Do not cook with Teflon-coated pans—there is toxins cooked into your food. Make sure that you store your leftovers and food in glass jars to avoid plastic toxins from contaminating your food.

Cleaning supplies also need to be detoxed. See the list provided. My favorite cleaning supplies, as I shared, is H20 at Home. Please refer to the back of the book, where you can purchase this product.

Have your water tested for chlorine. Reduce toxic body care products. See the list provided.

We have covered liver, gut, and hormonal detox in the other chapters. Please refer to them for guidance.

One last huge detox is of our emotional triggers. In order to cover that, we need to understand the meridian system a little bit better. We can sometimes uncover triggers when we look at our body and its restrictions. To be able to relieve past traumas in the body, we need to take a closer look at the Chinese meridian system. It is in this area we will be able to determine what structures in our body hold our discomfort and cause us to have emotional triggers.

Let's take a closer look at the body and the muscular structures in relation to the fascial lines and the Chinese traditional meridian lines. As I mentioned briefly, meridians traverse and go through the body. Each meridian has a partner, which is it's opposite. It balances out the energy that is traveling through the body. There are muscles of opposing forces that balance out the fascial lines that travel through the body.

When we look closer at how the body holds onto the tension from past traumas, and if we analyze deeply fascial structures, the meridians, and the muscles, we may be able to understand how we hold emotional triggers. For example, the emotion of grief. We may feel tightness in areas of the front of the chest and arms. Grief is expressed and is the emotion that is revealed in the yin lung meridian and the yang large intestine meridian. Together, these meridians hold the emotion of grief. I want to explain it further. I will break down the emotional components that we suffer from that may cause us to have certain tightness in the body.

I will start by going over the depths of the meridian system. There are six depths that correlate to an emotion. I will go over the depths, and I will include each meridian couple. These will be the areas in the body that hold tension or trauma from the past. I will explain which depth correlates to an emotion and explain where the fascial lines of tightness are in that depth. I will share behaviors, physical limitations, and/or illnesses that could be present in the body.

The first depth in the meridian system that will hold trauma in the body that I will share with you is the emotion of worry. The meridians involved in this depth are the stomach, which is the yang energy, and the spleen, which is yin energy. The stomach's emotional capacity is sympathy and compassion. Its fascial line is the superficial frontal spiral line, which traverses down the front of the body and twists through the body. Symptoms of discomfort that you may feel in the body might be lower leg pain, muscle pain, asthma, allergies, digestive problems, sweet cravings, irregular eating patterns, and gluttony. The spleen meridian is a yin energy. Its emotions are sympathy, self-love, and care for others.

Physical characteristics and symptoms that you may suffer from are asthma, allergies, diabetes, and increased sympathetic activity and stimulation. The first depth's emotions are worry, and rumination. You may experience your thoughts running in circles, feelings of being unloved, or low self-confidence. When this depth becomes unbalanced, we have a difficult time with digestive problems, weight gain, eating disorders, pancreas problems, skin disorders, and suffering from burnout.

The second depth: The emotion is grief. When you're sad for prolonged periods, this can cause your meridians to become sluggish and blocked. The two meridians that compromise the second depth are the lung meridian, which is yin energy, and the large intestine, which is yang energy. The fascial line is the deep frontal fascial line. Physical characteristics or symptoms include inability to take a breath, suffering from chronic bronchitis, asthma, and colds. A blockage in these meridians, again, is from the emotion of grief, sadness, and disappointment. If one is suffering from those emotions, they are impacting this meridian. You will have tightness in the front of the arms and in the chest.

The third depth: The emotion is anger. The meridians include the gallbladder and the liver meridians. The liver is the helper and has mental clarity and inspiration to act and gives us energy. The physical symptom is vision problems. Psychologically, there is anxiousness, codependency, and over-dependent behaviors. The liver fascial lines are the deep frontal line. The gallbladder, on the other hand, is the decision maker and can focus and plan. The fascial lines are the lateral fascial line. The psychological concern is fear. The physical symptoms include difficulty digesting fat, burping, gas, migraine headaches, and lower back pain. The third depth, again, is about anger and hardening of the thoughts, and feelings of frustration may consume you.

The fourth depth: The emotion is fear. The meridians involved in this depth are the bladder, which is the yang energy force, and the kidney meridian. The bladder meridian's emotion is as a performer. Its fascial lines are the posterior spiral line and superficial back lines. The physical symptoms when you start to have problems in this meridian are arthritis, ear infections, thyroid problems, frequent urination, bone disorders, and balance issues. The psychological concerns are anxiousness and narcissistic behaviors. The kidney is the other meridian in this depth, and it is a union energy. Its emotional trait is the comedian. The fascial lines are the deep frontal line. Physical symptoms can include low back pain, sciatica, shoulder pain, arthritis, ear infections, thyroid problems, incontinence, and menopausal symptoms.

The fifth depth: The emotion is pretense or trying too hard. The meridians are the small intestine and the heart meridian. The emotional trait of the small intestine is the artist. The fascial lines are the deep arm lines. The physical symptoms that you may see are abdominal bloating, warts, and shoulder problems. The psychological concern is anxiety. The heart meridian is in this depth. Its emotional trait is love. The fascial line is the superficial front line. The physical symptoms of this depth are mid-back and rib pain and tightness, pain in the shoulder, and carpal tunnel symptoms. The psychological concerns are the person may want to avoid situations and people and may suffer from forgetfulness. Physical symptoms are sleep disorders, insomnia, and circulation problems.

The six depth: The emotion is life-force, which is the feeling between the spirit the physical. The sixth depth meridians are the diaphragm meridian, which is yin, and the umbilicus meridian, which is yang energy. The emotional trait is hoping to find meaning in life. Psychological concerns are trust and impulsiveness. Physical symptoms are hormonal imbalance, night sweats, joint pain, shoulder and arm pain, ringing in the ears, and ear infection. Further physical symptoms include heart rate irregularities, blood pressure irregularities, hot flashes, excessive thirst, and possibly insulin resistance.

In order to relieve past trauma, we need to gently stretch and strengthen the injured fascia and meridian lines. Postures will impact how the brain interprets our state of being and its emotion. When we suffer from trauma, our body's fascia holds this information in it. The body and the brain talk to one another. The brain may try to hide or ignore the trauma if it is too difficult for it to process it. In these situations, we may not remember a traumatic incident. The body, however, remembers the event and signals the limbic system. Have you ever been in a situation that you felt a weird body response, like your hair on your back curling or you started to breath rapidly? That is what happens when your body sends a signal to the brain from the fascial lines. It stimulated the autonomic nervous system, and you don't even know why. Your body has memory stored in the fascia. It will stimulate the brain and the amygdala.

Studies have shown that by changing the posture, some of the trauma of PTSD can be relieved. Association of participation in a mindfulness program with measures of PTSD, depression and quality of life in a veteran sample "Journal of clinical psychology/ vol 68, issue 1. This study shows promising results of performing simple mindful changes to the body postures that can relieve some of the past trauma stored in the body. Recently, a new book that was just released by yoga instructor Eddie Stern—who is based in Brooklyn, New York—called One Simple Thing: A New Look at the Science of Yoga and How it Can Transform Your Life.

My husband was only able to reduce his trauma and gain his life back in part because of yoga and an anti-inflammatory diet, which helped to reduce the inflammation on his brain. You see, about six years ago, he was brutally assaulted and left for dead. He was beaten in the head, body, and neck. The brain injury affected his balance, vision, and sense of safety. He initially could not walk a straight line without falling to the right. He was fearful, angry, emotional, and depressed.

He is such a wonderful man. He is always so supportive of my adventures. When I started my yoga business, Balance Beyond the Mat, he said he would participate to help me kick off the classes. Little did I know how much it would help him. He started to not be fearful. He was able to sit in a busy place without his back against the wall. He could walk and stand on one leg, and his headaches were reducing. He was breathing with ease and not with fear. It has been six years and he is back to his profession, loving his life, and is able to laugh and relax without fear.

Best client ever.

When we move through yoga poses, we connect our mind to our body with our breath. Our breath controls the reaction of the autonomic nervous system, and as we stretch the tightened fascial lines and the meridians of that trauma, we can release the emotional blockages. Please check out my website and my webinar, "Yoga with Meridians," for actual poses and classes to take. Here are just a few quick stretches you can look up to gently help yourself.

At this time, I will share with you different yoga poses-asanas that will help to stretch the different emotional depths in the body.

The first depth is of the emotion to worry, the meridians are the stomach and the spleen. The yoga poses or asanas for the stomach are the twisted pigeon, downward-facing dog, forward bend, child's pose, plow, boat, wide-angle pose, wide-angle leg pose, and head-to-knee pose.

The second depth is of the emotion for grief, the meridians are the lung and large intestine. The yoga poses: half Lord of the Fishes, sage pose, reclining twists, revolved triangle, revolved extended side angle, angle pose, extended side angle pose, cow, cow face pose, eagle, and tree are also good stretches for these areas

The third depth is the emotion of anger, the meridians are the liver and the gallbladder. The yoga poses that are good for this are post triangle pose, lateral plank, half moon, extended side angle pose, extended triangle pose, revolved head-to-knee pose, child pose with your body side tilted to the left and then back to neutral, side child pose with your body side tilted to the right, and sun salutations. Asanas for the liver meridian are crescent moon, bridge pose, bow, and camel.

The fourth depth is the emotion of fear, the meridians are the kidney and the bladder. Yoga poses to help relieve this emotion are down dog, child, forward fold, and head-to-knees.

The fifth depth is the emotion of trying too hard or pretense, the meridians are heart and small intestine. The yoga poses are the one-legged royal pigeon pose and camel pose. Be cautious with these poses, especially if you have a sitting job and you have a tightened psoas muscle. These exercises will gently stretch the psoas muscle. On my website, I explain the importance of maintaining a healthy psoas muscle. It is a muscle that connects from your spine to your leg. It also attaches to the diaphragm. This muscle reacts to the stress in our body because of its attachment to the diaphragm.

A quick story of a past client. She was suffering from the inability to take a breath for about a year. She had many tests, trying to determine if she suffered from heart and lung complications. All tests came out normal. She came to me wanting to see if I could help her breathe better. She reported weight gain, stress at home due to her husband's illness, and pain in the mid-back and chest. After reviewing her foundational foods group, I noticed she enjoyed sitting and doing puzzles, and she also did a lot of furniture painting as a hobby. She was in a flexed position most of her day. I found that her right diaphragm was weak, and her right psoas muscle was in spasm. A few quick gentle stretches for her home exercise program and some strengthening exercises for her diaphragm helped her recover and achieve her goals within six weeks.

The sixth depth the emotions of life force, the meridians are diaphragm and the umbilicus. The yoga asana, corpse pose. Okay, this seems like a simple pose. This pose, if you are not familiar with it, is just lying flat on your back on a yoga mat on a hard surface. I cannot stress how important this pose is to do every day. Think about your day. You are flexed, sitting, bending over a desk, and bending forward over a task…. Rarely do we stretch our bodies out flat and straight. I know you may say, "Well, I lay in bed on my back." Not the same. Our beds are soft. They collapse at the heaviest section of our body—for women, the hips; for men, the chest—both of which flex the spine.

Every client of mine must be able to lie on the floor, stretch, breathe, and relax the tightened flexors of the body. I know what you are thinking: "It is too hard to get up off the floor. My hips or knees will not let me...." I am here to tell you what happens if you fall. Are you going to lay there until someone finds you? If you have a difficult time transferring from the floor to standing, or you have a spinal condition that restricts you from lying in a full neutral spine, I encourage you to research a physical therapist in your area and learn the proper methods for this transfer, or if it is okay for you to perform based on your spinal changes.

Ten minutes a day on the floor, breathing with the diaphragm, will help you to stretch out the tightened front muscles of your body and release toxic, tightened muscles of not only the fascia but emotional triggers of sadness and depression. When we are sad, our body goes into a slumped, shoulder-flexed position. Think about what the fascia tells our brain. "Slumped shoulders. I am sad...."

Now, you have the knowledge to detox your fascial lines and emotional blockages. It is amazing how powerful this can be. Not only will your body feel so much better, but also you will be able to think more clearly and your breath will come easier.

I enjoyed working with a mother of two teenagers once. She was a single mother. She suffered from a great amount of stress and financial burdens. She worked at a retail store. She enjoyed her job, but sometimes felt like customers dumped their crap on her. She was trying to raise her kids to be healthy and more self-confident in their life. As you can guess, we addressed some of her foundational food groups and finances. Her career needed some adjustments. When I evaluated her journal, I noticed that she was purchasing coffee drinks five days a week at four to five dollars each for each of them and purchasing dinners out three nights a week. Money was leaving her home for restaurants. Now, of course, I am a strong believer of being as great as I possibly can ninety percent of the time. Ten percent of the time, my angel wings are off. We adjusted some of the financial burdens of going out to one time per week, either a coffee or a dinner, one or the other.

This alleviated some of her financial burden, but made her feel squeezed to cook more at home. After I went through her pantry and detoxed the foods that caused her to crave processed food and junk food, she stopped purchasing boxed items. She did purchase an Instant Pot and a strong blender that could make vegetable sauces and dressing from fresh veggies and fruits. I encouraged her to cook on her days off, make sauces, and make her own fast food prep items at home.

I finally encouraged her to think about each customer on their journey. Some people are just difficult because of where they are in their life journey. I have a saying that I use with my kids: "You cannot rationalize with crazy, be nice to mean, or save someone that loves being a victim." It will waste your time and effort. I encourage my clients to wrap an invisible mirror around their body that faces out to who they deal with. Somehow, this protects our spirit and causes the other person to see themselves in their full glory.

Once we were able to establish some minor changes, my client's stress went down, her finances improved, and she was able to enjoy her kids without feeling financially strapped. She learned not to take other people's journey on her life, and, no big surprise, her body stopped being in a fight, flight, and/or fear state and she lost her weight. She did start doing movement and yoga in addition to eating proper foods to implement her weight loss and physical body health. She was so fun to work with. We still work together to keep those nasty triggers at bay.

It is starting to get fun, right? You learn so much of what causes your body to get angry and gain weight. Who knew we were doing this to our body? Once we detox our pantry, stop the uncontrollable cravings caused from processed foods, change our mind thoughts and talk, detox people that are not challenging and loving us to be and become our best, and get rid of the poisons in our environment that make our liver work so hard and throw off our hormones, we do not have to work so hard to lose the weight and feel better physically.

The next chapter will incorporate what we need to do when we know better.

----------------------------------- ✗ ✗ ✗ -----------------------------------

Chapter 10
What We Know Now

"What you do is up to you.
What I do is up to me.
What is going to be,
Is up to me."
— **Aunt Ruth Gummersall-Hansen-Holt**

Step 7

*I*sn't is surprising to realize that we have more than food that feeds us? What we place on our plates is only a small part that contributes to our health. The foundational food groups that we analyzed should make a little impression on how your life is moving. If you have found yourself running from place to place, job to job, and task to task, it might be time to ask yourself why you do it. I know it seems like you do not have a choice, but maybe you do. I know that life is busy. It can seem like there is no time for yourself, but it is up to you to make it happen. It is only you that can take the little steps to make the changes. There may be some hidden reasons why you keep running. Hopefully we have been able to uncover some of the more important areas of your life that you will start to work to have your dream life. Review your dream picture and go toward it. Remember on the way to make the choice that will help you achieve this dream.

When we are children, we suffer from triggers. The triggers can be positive or negative. Either way, they cause us to remember an event that can transform us. We may not remember the event, but our brain does. The brain will store it in the body, and when something is like the event, it is brought to us again. Our body will tell the brain, and we will adjust as we did when the initial event occurred. This may be one of the reasons that we try to do so much.

Life isn't fun if we collapse on the coach from exhaustion. When the triggers are pulled and we start to doubt our self-worth, we cause our body to fail. We can only do so much. It isn't our responsibility to make everything happen. It is our responsibility to live our life with intent and purpose. But when we run ourselves physically and emotionally down, we do ourselves no good. We harm ourselves.

There are times in our life that we get caught up in just doing. We stop enjoying. It is important to uncover why we slipped into the "just doing" in life. At that time, we need to look at the triggers in our life that caused our ego to shift from our inner beauty to what the outer world needs.

When I finally realized that I was a beautiful light, from a divine source, my divine source is God. Yours can be nature, an atom, or the universe—it doesn't matter. It is your source and that's what's important. It is something that you believe in.

If you think about this, our divine source wants us to have health and prosperity. It only wants the best for us. It doesn't want us in pain or to see us struggle. We were created out of love. Let me ask you a question. If you have something that you created, a child, or a piece of art, clay sculpture or painting—do you want to see it be destroyed, or self-destruct, get hurt, or made to feel worthless? No. You want it to feel love for itself and see how beautiful it is.

What makes us stop believing in ourselves and our self-worth is not because of our creator. It is because of the ego, or the experiences that were presented to us. The soul, true conscious, or the inner being is beautiful. It was created for pure love. What prevented us from achieving our ultimate self is our ego and our environment, like the Petri dish and its different cultural mediums that changed the same cell into bone, skin, or muscle. The petri dish is no different than our environment and our journey that we traveled.

This journey taught us to talk terribly to ourselves, which damages our bodies and our beliefs of who we are. The people we surround ourselves with, the foods that we eat, the environment we stay in—that is our petri dish. Bruce Lipton writes in *The Biology of Belief* that we can change our environment for the better. If our environment can make us chose poorly, once we know better, we can decide for the better by changing our environment for the better. What we take in to surround ourselves with should be for the better. His petri dishes of the cells change, and we can too.

Now, it was said that fifty percent of our emotional responses to things are from our genetics and fifty percent is from our environment. I think this is a little bit funny because, if I think about my genetics, I understand a little bit more why I worry so much. I think about my mom, who was the twelfth of thirteen kids in the Great Depression. She constantly was trying to always be of use. I think that affected me because I always feel like, for me to be loved or wanted, I need to work hard. My father was a prisoner of war. He felt if he didn't provide what was expected of him, he would be killed. Fifty percent of that, no matter what I do, is part of me. No wonder I have a difficult time with a little bit of anxiety. However, I can change or rewrite what my thoughts and life are by being mindful of what I surround myself with.

Now, the triggers in our life are the materials in our petri dish. We will grow to become what we experience. Remember one of the examples I used earlier in the book, my father saying to me, "Don't be an ornament?" That impacted my fascia, and I am constantly trying to work all the time to earn my keep. I have to constantly talk to myself to change this belief. When I feel the fear in my gut, I realize what it is from. I change the message in my brain. The journey we walk determines our biology. What we say to ourselves creates a memory in our brain. We play it over and over. To some extent, we play it to protect us. It hurts, and if it hurts, we want to avoid it.

Now, you may say that this is not anything that relates to you, but if you try to do everything for everyone else and not take care of yourself, what message is that? Everyone else is more important than you…Maybe we should consider why you do it. I know you want to lose weight, but if you keep going at this pace, you will wear yourself out. You have one body. It can take this for so long, and then it will stop.

What are some of your triggers that may have made your life turn out the way it has? The extra weight was caused in part from the stress you underwent. The foundational food groups that have not served your soul will cause you to have inflammation in your body from all the low-grade chronic stress. I encourage you to just slow down and take some time to say, "Is this working for me?" I think that sometimes we just try to please everyone else and not ourselves. We try to make everyone else happy, and we suffer. But what I want to try to impart on you is that you are important, and when you feel that you are worthy, your brain will reward your body and the stress will slow down. Take the time to enjoy your life. It is truly up to you. I gave you the tools to change what your body is trying to tell you. It is up to you to make the change. Be kind to yourself. If one day you did a great job and the next day you did not, don't punish yourself. The words you say to yourself are just as toxic as the processed food we learned about.

When the student is ready, the teacher appears. If this book doesn't speak to you, you were not ready for me to appear. I am here to share with you what helped me stop the weight gain and the self-destructive workloads. I realized that I am worthy. I am enough. I want you to realize now, after you looked at your life in its entirety, that you are worthy of a beautiful life and not just a life that you run in. It is time for you to take the time to enjoy your life.

I truly believe, deep down, all we want is to be loved, receive appreciation, and be respected. Somehow, we learned to get those from behaving according to what helped us survive in the past. I was primed from an early ancestry to be a superwoman. To overcome something hard served my superpowers. I received attention when I said it was too much and was able to make it happen. I was rewarded with attention. But does this serve my body now?

The ego will do the behavior that serves its purpose, but it may not serve the body and your inner conscious.

Listen to your body. Learn to feel where it is talking to you, what it is telling you, and what it wants. If you can't decipher what your body is saying, then where are you restricted? Stretch those areas gently with yoga. Breathe and connect the brain to the body with your breath. The truth is, when you are ready to accept how truly important you are, you will take the time to take care of you.

I listened to self-help messages my entire life, and when I was open to receive the message, I became aware of a little bit more of who I was. The universe or your source will give you messages along the way if you open your heart up to receiving them. Your true purpose will be presented to you. The weight is just another message from your body that something is off-balance. The way you feed your foundational foods may be contributing to the weight gain, but more importantly, it is contributing to your health. As you feed your foundational food groups with the right thought and actions, your body will respond, and your life will change. You will no longer try to be the person who tries to do everything for everyone else and not for yourself.

Chapter 11

When We Know Better, We Do Better

"People need to wake up and stop sleeping through their life. It's like waiting to have sex when you're old."

– Warren Buffett

Step 8

I have taught you a lot up to this point. Throughout the book, you were given reasons for why the body reacts the way it does. Now, we will recap and explain a few of the step you can do to eliminate the body's reactions. We will address stress, food, avoiding toxins, the crowding out food plan which was introduced to me by the Institute of Integrative Nutrition. We will also address how we can take a pause to take care of ourselves, use our calendar, and ask for help. We need to clean up the toxins, and that includes Wi-Fi.

One of the ways we can decrease the stress our body suffers from is to decrease brain stress and improve your repeated history messages that the brain continues to spin. A great way to reduce the stress that we're experiencing is to perform mindful activities, such as take a walk and really be present with what you see, feel, hear, and smell, use all of your senses to acknowledge what is happening around you. Another mindful activity can be just sit and use your senses to be aware of your present state. Be present in the moment.

In order to get the brain out of the hyperactive chronic stress, we need to do stress-relieving activities. Another stress-relieving activity that is shown to decrease the autonomic nervous system stimulation and the fight or flight is meditation for ten to fifteen minutes. Meditation can help to reduce stress on the brain.

A simple meditation can be one that is placing your focus on your breath. Inhale on a count of six and exhale to a count of eight. Count the respirations as you exhale. Continue for thirty-six breaths. Remember, you are counting on the exhalation. If you lose count, start over. This type of meditation can be done while waiting in a car, at your desk, or practically anywhere. Your focus is on your breath and counting. If you drift and worry about something, come back to the counting.

The important aspect in this is the exhalation must be longer than the inhalation. Fear is produced in our body when we do short quick breaths or hold our breath. This signals to the brain that we need to produce more oxygen. The brain will respond with stimulation of the autonomic nervous system.

In order to reduce stimulation in the amygdala and hippocampus, we need to activate the prefrontal cortex. We also need to decrease the autonomic nervous system's fight or flight reaction. The goal is to try and stimulate the parasympathetic system, which is rest and digest.

Some ways to do that is learning a new skill. Learning a new skill activates the prefrontal cortex. Focus on a task, hold a posture as in yoga, try to balance on one foot, do a puzzle—anything that you must focus your attention on performing.

We now know how to clean up the diet, avoid processed foods, and avoid foods that contain pesticides. Go green and organic, avoid toxins around your home, and avoid added sugars, white starchy foods, trans-fats, antibiotics, and hormones in your food. Eat regular meals, especially breakfast. Try to follow the Chinese meridian clock. Do try to eat within one hour of waking.

The portion size of your meal is simply this. How much did you say you wanted to weigh in the goals section of our process? When you dish your plate up, is it to feed that size of a person? If you want to be 120 pounds, does your plate look like it's for someone who weighs 120 pounds? Is it heaped up to feed a 200-pound person? You know this! I will not let you kid yourself anymore. Eat the weight you want to be.

What you put on your plate is also important. Your vegetables portion is half your plate, your protein is the size of your palm, your grains are the size of your cupped fingers, and your fats should be about the size of your thumb.

Space your meals five to six hours apart. If you have blood sugar issues, a bedtime snack is okay. Avoid simple carbohydrates, though. Try to avoid eating between dinner and breakfast, and drink plenty of water.

Eat high-quality proteins, fats, and fiber. Utilize the crowd out policy. Try to eat your largest portion of the meal to be plant-based. Consume the colors of the rainbow with your vegetables. Next, eat protein and then a good-quality grain. Crowd out the fatty foods with the good. Eat more veggies. Eat more of these to fill you up.

Crowd out the consumption of alcohol and caffeine with water. Try to drink a glass of water after each cup of coffee. In the morning, I have a glass of sixteen ounces of water by my bed with a lemon slice squeezed in it. In the morning, I drink this first thing in order to help my stomach acids get ready for the day of food.

Include in your diet omega-3s, EPAs, and DHA sources. These are wild caught fatty fish, avocados, walnuts, cheese, seeds, hemp hearts. If you do not eat this type of food, make sure to take a good supplement.

Remember, we established a destination in the beginning of this book. You outlined what you wanted your life to look like. There is a plan, a roadmap, and a destination that you travel to. Plan on doing that with everything in our life, and that includes meal prep.

Every week, I prep for my meals. You must to have a plan for meal prep. It's the same as the picture. If we don't have a destination of where we are going, we will just float. I act like my house is a fast food restaurant. Fast food restaurants do well because food is prepared before the guest comes in. They are fast. It's unfortunate they use so much processed terrible food; however, we don't have to do that at our house. On my days off, I take the time to cook the meat for the week, so if I want to have chicken, beef, poultry, and pork, it is ready for the week. I also plan on my days off to prep my produce and my vegetables. I wash them, chop them, and prepare them. I then place them in a glass Pyrex dish and I have them stacked in the refrigerator for easy access.

I can now have a stir-fry, a salad, or a side dish. It is fast food ready in my refrigerator. I may cook a pot of beans, black beans, or garbanzo beans, and I place them in mason jars in the fridge. I use them through the week for salads or sides. I cook up a large batch of quinoa, or brown rice, or wild rice for more grain.

When you prepare your food, your food acts like a fast food restaurant at your home. Meals are easy to put together. Remember me. I was coming in at 10:00 p.m. and eating fast food and drinking wine. If I can do it, so can you.

Remember to take a pause repeatedly though out the day. Stop and breathe. Perform a meditative breathing in which you inhale on a count of six and exhale on a count of seven. The exhales always need to be longer in order to stimulate the parasympathetic nervous system.

Let's think a little bit about this. When you are scared, what is the first thing you do? You hold your breath. Holding your breath notifies the amygdala. Exhale, breath slowly, and belly breathe using your diaphragm. This will stimulate the parasympathetic system, or the rest and digest response.

Create clear boundaries with you time and priorities. This is one of the biggest obstacles that people don't do. If you've ever noticed, women are particularly terrible at this. They continue to take more onto their plate, and this causes them to not have enough time to perform all the activities or jobs that they placed on themselves initially well. The running cycle needs to stop. If we, as women, are unable to complete all of the tasks, we feel uneasy, and stress starts. Trying to do too much also causes us to feel like we don't do anything well. Stress happens again. Take a pause- remember.

Your calendar is your new shield. Take it everywhere. Always document more time than you think you need for your commitments. The worst feeling is when we have scheduled ourselves so tightly that we are late to each appointment. I also want you to be realistic about the time it takes to do an activity. How many times have we said we can do something, but we run into a snag: our computer doesn't work, the car is out of gas, and the kids call and want you to wash their sport clothes. Planning for these interruptions is a way to decrease your stress.

Also, be prepared when someone asks you to do something. Take a pause think about it. If you're not sure you want to do it, don't feel guilted into agreeing to do it. Remember, you need to put the oxygen mask on you first, not anyone else.

Ask for help. Some of the old triggers we carry around make us feel like if we don't do everything, we aren't doing a good job. Try to ask for help cleaning the house. Also, take advantage of the shopping at the convenient market system where you can order your groceries online and pick them up. Someone will come out and deliver them to your car. Utilize some of the professions available, like cleaning services or lawn care. If you can't afford it… teach your kids. The ripple effect of us doing it all is that we have kids that don't know how to cook, clean, wash their clothes, or fix their cars. We are enabling our children.

By now, you know that trying to do it all is making you gain weight and start a decline in health. Realize and limit what you're doing. Crowding out when we eat is important, but we can do that with activities that cause us stress. Crowd out the stressful events in your life. If you feel like you're running from place to place to place, take one of those objects off your plate, delegate, and move to a more restful position.

There are a lot of restorative activities that you can do. One that I like to do to wind down at night is to walk barefoot in the grass. This is called earthing, and it grounds us the Earth's pole. I do it for thirty minutes. There are studies that show that this helps to relieve some of the stress in our body.

Clean up the wi-fi time. In one study in the *Environmental Research*, wi-fi and other electromagnetic field exposures were found to increase oxidative stress to our bodies and increase the stress response, causing hormone changes, teste and sperm dysfunction, cellular DNA damage, endocrine changes, and calcium overload. All of these are caused from having the electric current near our bodies for prolonged periods of time. Do not plug your phone or computer up in your bedroom.

Remember the days when the phone that was plugged in didn't ring after nine p.m.? If it did, it was an emergency. We discussed toxic wi-fi. Stop looking at T.V., Facebook, Snapchat, and Instagram until all hours of the night. The blue rays affect your sleep. Try to bring back some of those old rules of no social media or phone calls after nine p.m. It will take so much stress out of your body. Before you fall asleep, you will be surprised.

Think back about the days when you were your happiest. Try to reengage in those hobbies. Learn a new skill. Let your mind think about something to learn instead of worry about. Make sure you take time to have a social network that feeds your soul. We need to have our friends and a time to relax and have bonding time with people that get us and have the same values as we do. Remember to get rid of the toxic people. People that suck our energy doesn't help us to feel good. Surround yourself with people that accept what you are and what you can do. Surround yourself with the people that make you want to grow and be better as a person because that is how they live. We tend to become what we are around. Make sure the people in your life fit into what you established as your dream life. If they do not, they are not helping you to achieve your health goals.

When you start your day every morning, when you get up, you have a choice to look at the day as a bright new day or a terrible day. You have the choice to think about positive things or negative things.

Every morning I wake up with anxiety, I feel that I'm not going to get everything done on my list in the day. I look at my list of events that I have to attend, and I look at the activities that I'm supposed to perform. I look at what is happening around my environment. My mind starts to race, my heart rate goes up, and I am scared. But, every day, I learned that I must control this fear. I place myself in a position of comfort. I either listen to the waterfall or I watch the hummingbirds outside my window. I do a simple breathing to stop my sympathetic nervous system from overreacting. I inhale, and I must exhale longer. I try to stretch out my body so that I'm not in a flexed position and release the tightened fascia and meridians. I do some gentle soft talking to myself. I have a mantra I say to myself that grounds me to who I am and what my purpose is in this life. This may sound crazy, but every morning, I feel like there is this negative committee in my head that says I'm not going be able to make it through the day. This committee in my head, the thoughts that run around crazily and try to make me feel scared, I named it. It is called the Bull-Crap Committee. I've named every member of the committee. I have a Negative Nancy, a What-If Wanda, a Jealous Jane, an Insecure Ida, a Fearful Fred, and an Angry Andy. This is a big committee. It continues with Shameful Sarah, Sad Sally, Victim Vicky, Not-Good-Enough Nick, Stressed-Out Sam, Anxious Annie, and Ruminating Rhonda. When they chatter at me about whatever their section is to bring up, and when it makes me feel like I'm not going to make it through the day, I fire them. I fire them out of my brain. I say, "You're fired," and I think about something else. If it was Jealous Jane that I fired, I think about Grateful Greta, and I try to review all the good things that happened in my morning. If it's Negative Nancy, I think about Hopeful Holly. This is my way of trying to control some of my anxiety.

My brother Frank suffered from anxiety from the age of nine. He was never able to control the fear, and I believe that is one of the reasons why he died at age fifty-seven. Try to control your fear or whatever you worry about. Use your breath to connect your mind and your body and control the sympathetic system. This will shut it down and, with your longer exhalations, you stimulate the rest, digest, and relaxation response. Please be present in the now. Think about only your breathing. Realize everything will be okay, give your brain a fact to focus on, not a what-if. Just connect your brain to your body with your breath.

Each morning, I listen to my body and the areas of tightness that I feel in the different chakras, the fascial lines, and the meridians. I gently stretch out on my mat and breathe into each area. I know you don't feel like you have the time to do this, but what is the price you pay if you don't do it? Stress all day? I take the time to do this now. I didn't used too. I used to race out the door. Now, I get up at least ninety-five minutes before I even must get ready to leave the house. Find the time to move your body and your heart. Make the movement enjoyable: walking, dancing, biking, hiking—something each day where you take your joints throughout the entire range of motion. If you do not use it, you will lose it. This includes your muscles, heart, lungs, and joints. I can't tell you how much this improved my life. My life is so much calmer.

Plan your life and have a destination. Everything that you do should move you to your big picture, not only for weight loss but also in how you act every day, how you relate to your body, and how you listen to your body. If you have soreness in your neck, what did you do yesterday that caused that soreness? If you couldn't prepare for your meals, what can you do that's healthy quickly? I know there will be days that you seem to get derailed. Here is where you stop beating yourself up and sabotaging the next day. It is okay to have a cheat day. I try to do the ninety/ten rule. I try to do the best I can for my mind, my body, and my spirit ninety percent of the time. Do I enjoy the ten percent? You bet. But what I have stopped doing to myself that I did in the past was I stopped the negative talk to myself, which I believe causes weight to stay on more than food. I now think about what I want my life to be like at the end of my life. I want to be able to walk and feel light and healthy.

If you want that picture in your life that you established as a goal in the second step of this process, it is up to you to show up for your life.

It is time for you to live, be healthy, and have a great life. Stop waiting for the last days of your life when it is too late.

Your calendar is your new superpower. Use it wisely. Black out times in your day for yourself. I know this seems unrealistic. I understand that you have children, commitments, jobs, and people, and someone's always after you to do something. But, if you don't take care of yourself, no one else will. If you don't respect your time, no one else will respect your time. You model the behavior of how you want people to treat you. Take your calendar and use it wisely. Use it to give borders and boundaries around yourself so that you can take care of yourself. It is time to show up for your life.

---------------------------------- ✗·✗·✗ ----------------------------------

Chapter 12
Yeah, But…

"It is health that is real wealth and not pieces of gold and silver."
– Mahatma Gandhi

J he life we live in is stressful. We push ourselves to work more, do more, and juggle more as women. How many hats do you wear? We, as women, we wear at least six hats, actually more like ten or twelve. We are mom, wife, home manager, tutor, employee, taxi service, chef, and groundskeeper, not to mention laundry service, nurse, coach, friend, and support system. With all these hats we wear, we run on high. Even with all those tasks, we still have another hurdle to leap. We not only do too much in our foundational food groups, but also, we feed our bodies toxins and unhealthy food. Our food sources are depleted, and our bodies cannot break down the chemicals we poison ourselves with. We poison ourselves with processed foods not because we want to, but because we didn't realize how they damaged our body.

For years, I yo-yo dieted. I raced from place to place and spread myself too thin. I accepted every task assigned to me. I tried to please everyone. I was the person that felt like I truly was responsible for everyone's happiness. I accepted every demand even when I didn't want to. I felt like I wouldn't be liked if I didn't do what people wanted me to do. I felt like I would let them down. I felt like it was up to me to make everything right. What I realized is that I am responsible only for myself and my happiness. I am not responsible to others to make their life happy. That is their responsibility. I learned that I do not need to accept this responsibility. I detoxed my life of people that want me to make them happy. It isn't my job. I do the best job I can wherever I am. I show up for my life.

I believe that we truly want to be loved for who we are. But, as we travel through life, we stumble. We doubt ourselves. Our self-talk and our self-belief of who we are impact our health. When we continue to rush and place demands on our bodies, we will slowly fail. Trying to do everything as a woman when we truly are the center of our house only depletes our body. We are the center of the family. Our children come to us for all their needs. Our husbands need us to help them be confident and successful. We are at the center, yet, when we also become the person who climbs to the top of the corporate ladder, we lose our sense of self. We want to be amazing in every task we attempt. We can only do so much.

I want to share a story of some of my past clients. It truly shows what may happen if we chose to ignore what our body is saying to us.

When I was about twenty-seven years old, I met two wonderful women. It was very early in my career as a physical therapist, and I was impressed with two women that came through my door.

Valerie was a vivacious, outgoing, intelligent woman, and just seemed to have everything put together. She spoke highly of her family. She enjoyed trips with her family, and she enjoyed her life. She exercised daily, but not an exercise that she didn't enjoy. She was the person that turned me on to yoga.

She had three children, and she loved her husband so much. She did share that he would irritate her every once and awhile. She told me how he would try and overschedule their family. I remember asking her what she meant. She said he would overschedule or put too many events on the calendar. He would constantly put more activities on their calendar that would not fit. I giggled at that. At that time in my life, that was me. I didn't understand what she's talking about because I put too many things on my calendar all the time. What I noticed about Valerie was that she enjoyed her life. She enjoyed great food and had fun with her husband. She also enjoyed her children. They would ski, hike, and kayak. She had a great group of friends that she would go out with. Once a year, they planned an event that she travelled to with her girlfriends. They went to California.

Valerie did work, but she said that she would rather not have every trinket in order to have a life that she loved. She said it wasn't important to her to have the biggest house or the nicest car. She said that she would rather have financial freedom and not spend. Valerie was so impressive to me. I remember Valerie stating that her boss wanted her to accept a promotion at her job. I thought that sounded awesome. She turned it down because it would take away from her family life. She did not want to take on something that would cost her too much stress.

Jade was the on the opposite of the spectrum from Valarie. Jade would work many hours at work. She was the most successful woman in her corporation. She wore suits into the clinic and drove beautiful cars. She constantly talked about how she was flying to this place and doing this new adventure. She was constantly hosting parties and was so busy.

What I noticed about Jade is that she constantly was worried. Her calendar was completely booked. Every day had something on it. I remember asking Jade what her hobbies were. She said she didn't have time for hobbies. I remember asking Jade about her children, and she said with all the time at the office, she hardly ever saw them. I remember talking to her about her husband, and she said, "Well, I'm so busy. At night, when I get home, I just collapse on the couch. I don't have time to be intimate or to have fun. I just am working and trying to just survive. I want to make sure that my family is provided for."

I remember asking Jade if she had a social group or time for friends. She did not have time for them. She spent her time at work. Jade didn't exercise nor did she cook. I shared this story because I recently heard from both women. They are both approaching eighty-five years of age.

Valerie is still Valerie; she has a cropped haircut and it's just spicy. She is running around like she used to, socializing and enjoying her life. I asked her what she was doing recently, and she was flying to California for her eighty-fifth birthday. I asked her how her husband was, and she said he passed away, but she said that she had so many beautiful years with him. She was grateful. Valerie was running, moving, dancing, laughing, and enjoying her life still at eighty-five.

Later, I ran into Jade's daughter. It was a sad situation for me. She shared with me that her mom wasn't doing well, that she was in a nursing home. She developed Alzheimer's and was unable to breathe well. She was on oxygen 100 percent of the time. Jade didn't remember her family.

I thought for a moment about both women who I had so much respect for when I was twenty-seven years old, I thought of how they were at the top of the world when I met them years ago. Both of them were strong, independent women, but now one was in the nursing home and one was flying to California for her eighty-fifth birthday. I learned a lot that day. I realize that I wanted to be that person that was flying to California at eighty-five.

With my thirty years in the medical profession, this is a reoccurring theme. I witnessed beautiful, vivacious, strong women become ill and not live fully to the end of their life. They try to do it all and be it all for everyone. I watched them do everything for their family and not take time for themselves. Many of the women that I started my practice with returned to me for further help. I see some of them and they are tired and old, not in years but in health and function. The ones that didn't take the time for themselves, prioritize their family, prioritize their time, and surround themselves with good people were ill. The women who did take the time to take care of themselves were still skiing and traveling. They were functionally living with health.

It scares me to see how many of these amazing women deteriorated. Some of them suffer from autoimmune deficiencies, fibromyalgia, MS, Parkinson's, rheumatoid arthritis, and dementia. I believe we don't have a choice but to take care of ourselves. We owe it to our family and our society.

Our stress load is affecting our bodies. We have extra weight that bothers us and makes us feel less than we are. We suffer from hormonal imbalances, food toxicity, and sugar overload. Not only do we have to manage our foundational food groups, but with some of our food sources, we constantly damage our bodies.

I know that there are so many reasons you feel that you won't be able to stick with this program. I had the same reasons. I felt that everyone else was more important than I was. I suffered from weight gain, hair loss, and HPA axis dysfunction, also known as adrenal failure. I was in constant pain. I didn't think I was important enough to take care of myself, but then I realized, if I die, how will that help my family?

I started to learn about what was making me sick. I shared that in its entirety with you.

Please make the decision sooner rather than later to help yourself. It isn't only about helping yourself. It is about helping your children. Kids will do what you do. They will grow up to be exactly what you modeled. If you continue to rush and have no time to plan, that is what you will be teaching your children and their children. It will affect future generations. It seems like too big of a price to pay for you not to take the knowledge you learned and change your life and your family's life. I am always available to you. My website is www.suesealwellness.com also my e-mail address is SueSealWellness@gmail.com I know that your life and your children will benefit from your knowledge.

You are the beginning of a ripple. It is up to you to help yourself and show the future how to live to be beautiful and functional at the end of your life.

Chapter 13
You Did It

"Happiness is your birthright."
– Gabrielle Bernstein

$\mathcal{I}$ hope you've enjoyed this book and the description of my process to help you lose the weight and get rid of your spandex. By now, you should be able to get into your jeans and any clothes that are in your closet, but more importantly, you should have a better understanding of your body and your brain.

Through this book, I have discussed the different steps to health and weight loss. We learned about your gut health and what happens when we have an imbalance of our good gut bacteria to bad bacteria. Too much sugar and too much processed food injures the liver and the gut and disrupts the hormones. When there is a dys-biosis, or an imbalance, in the gut, we have inflammation in our body. That inflammation will damage to our cells, and our body will have illness and decreased strength and stamina.

I have discussed how stress can affect our hormones and cause an imbalance in our hormones, which, in turn, will start weight gain and inflammation. I have taught you how to re-structure your foundational food groups and help your gut heal. There are many wonderful foods out there that do help the gut stop the inflammation.

The eight steps, in summary, began with understanding where you are in the process of your life. You are busy—you take care of your children and your home. When you work, you run from task to task, and life just seems to get away from you.

I educated you and reviewed your foundational food groups and helped you realize that the foods that feed your soul and spirit are just as important as the foods that you feed your body. The foundational food groups consist of our social environment with our friends and how important it is to have a friend group that we know supports us and loves us. Our relationship with our husband or mate is important for us to feel loved, appreciated, and respected. The financial situation you are in, how it feeds us, does it give us security or a sense of fear. Your career and work also impact your health and your body.

Try to think about this from now on, about how important foundational food groups are. If the foundational food groups suffer, it will cause undue stress, which causes our body to react with stimulation of the autonomic nervous system.

Then, spiritually, we realized that the universe and our higher source have strength beyond ourselves, and that sometimes the environment we are in takes away the beauty of our inner self. I helped you realized that who you surround yourself with and the environment that we surround ourselves with contribute to our health, how we treat ourselves, and how we feel about ourselves.

It is important always to remember to optimize your nutrition to help balance your hormones and decrease the gut dys-biosis and the sugar intolerances. This, in turn, will help to reduce inflammation, help you lose weight, and gain a functional, healthy body.

Discussion of the past triggers in our lives that cause us to race and work beyond what our body can tolerate helped us to learn that we are worthy and that we can take the time to care for ourselves. Learning and controlling some of the triggers that we've had in the past can be relieved with Eastern medicine, gentle yoga, and the chakra system.

Stress management is important to stop the harmful imbalances in our bodies. Learn to take a pause and breathe. Slow down the negative voices in our heads. It is important for us to continue to think about what we are in this world as women. We are the ripple effect to our children and the society. When we rush and don't take care of ourselves, we model this behavior to our children. They, too, will do that, and with that comes illness for them. Take the time to love yourself. Breathe.

I am excited for the new steps you will be taking in your life. My wish for you is that you take the time to take care of yourself. I know it may seem like it's selfish, but it truly isn't. The steps you take now for your life will help you have a beautiful end of life. I took you from the spot of losing weight to the spot of knowing how to take care of your body. You can have the body of your dreams, not only now with the clothes fitting but also with the body that will take you into your older years.

When you are older, I want you to be able to enjoy every moment; to be at the end of your life and still be able to walk, smile, laugh, and dance; to be able to enjoy your grandchildren, hiking, strolling on the beach, and all the things that life has to offer for you. I know for a fact that what we do to our body today at our age affects how we will show up at the end of our lives. We witnessed that with the two women that impacted my life when I was younger: Valarie, vivacious and charismatic, moving and hiking up to her eighty-fifth birthday; and Jade, the other woman, for her eighty-fifth birthday who had done everything in her life to be that person for everyone else. I remember seeing her when I was young and how I thought that she was doing everything amazing. She was taking care of her job, her kids, her house, and her husband, and she was so busy. She was full of life then. But what I remember of Jade was that she was fearful and worried. She was trying so hard to keep up with all the jobs on her plate. She never gave any time to herself. She was the woman that said yes to the boss for the extra project, yes to the PTA to help at the functions, and yes to her husband that wanted to have company parties. She said yes to everyone but herself.

The other woman, Valarie, said no to the people that she didn't want in her life. She said yes to the people that filled her up, gave her happiness, and made her soul laugh. She took care of her body and listened to it. She ate proper foods and she had the greatest foundational groups surrounding her. She made the choice to have that foundational group that she chose, and she chose wisely. She didn't just let life happen to her. She chose her life and made it happen. What I want for you is to be Valerie, who still is enjoying life at eighty-five, jumping on planes and flying all over. She has her life because she chose to make her life what it is.

Oh, hey, remember Sara? The woman I spoke about at the beginning of the book? She has been with my program since I have been writing this book. I am happy to report that Sara has lost thirty-five pounds, is feeling less stressed, and is able to sleep at night. Better yet, she just told me yesterday, "I think that this is the first time in my life that I have enjoyed my life. I am not thinking of what I need to do every minute. I am living in the moment and enjoying each moment." Sara found that a gentle walking program, yoga stretches, and balancing work every day helped her body feel better. She also joined a dance group and is learning the salsa. She detoxed her life and loves her home and environment. For the first time since I have known her, she is laughing. I am the luckiest person in the world. I get to help people laugh and relax again.

That is my wish for you. I want you to enjoy your life now and in the future. I believe Gabrielle Bernstein is correct: "Happiness is our birthright." I want you to claim this. Take back your life.

I don't want to see you alone with your body broken in a retirement home because you can't take care of yourself. I want to see you having a great end of life, a functional end of life. You have all the tools to do it and, better yet, you have the tools to share with your children and your grandchildren that they will share with their children. It takes one step in the right direction, and you will be modelling a heathy future for your grandchildren. I know you don't want your grandchildren to be rushing and racing, trying to get everything done for everyone but themselves.

It only takes you to just realize that you have one body. It cannot be turned in for another one. We have one body. We can ignore it and let it fail, or we can listen to it and thrive. We are in control of our destination. We are in control of our life. We can choose to waste it or make it spectacular. What we do with our lives will ripple through our children. We need to teach our children how to take care of themselves, how to take care of their bodies, and how to respect their bodies so that they can have that beautiful end of life also.

We need to show up for our lives.

Disclaimer

The information in this book is not intended or implied to be a substitute for professional medical advice, diagnosis, or treatment. All content including text, graphics, images and information, contained in this book is for general educational and informational purposes only and may not be construed as medical advice. The information is not intended to replace medical advice offered by physicians. Please seek the advice of your medical physician prior to participation of any of the outlined actives or exercises found in this book. The author does not dispense medical advice or prescribe any techniques as a form of treatment for physical or emotional problems in this book and requires that you seek medical advice from a physician before proceeding with any information outlined in this book. In the event that you use any information in this book for yourself, the author assumes no responsibility for your actions

Acknowledgments

This book owes a great deal to my patients of the past. Many entered my life requiring my help, but continued to serve society beyond their ability, causing them to suffer from weight gain and health issues merely because they were trying to keep up with life. This book is for those people I've seen do their best without asking for much in return for themselves. It is because of these incredible people I realized they needed help realizing their greatness as who they are, to encourage them to understand that they are worthy regardless of what they do.

I am extremely thankful for Dr. Christiane Northrup for introducing me to understanding my body on a deeper level and for pointing me in the right direction to help myself become a healthier person. I am also very thankful to the Institute of Integrative Nutrition for the education I received that help me refine my understanding of diet and nutrition.

I am so grateful for the people who surround me and help me strive to be a better person. To my yogis, thank you for being the tribe that keeps me moving and breathing. To my "mom tribe," thank you for being such giving moms and for raising gorgeous children for our future. Thank you to my coworkers and friends at OSS MultiCare who with heart in hand, help clients achieve a functioning life.

I want to thank my brothers and sisters who have helped guide me to be who I am. To my parents, thank you for enlightening me to be my best and to never give up. And finally, thank you to my wonderful husband and children, who are the heart and soul of my being. Thank you for being who you are, and for being a part of my world.

Special Thank you to Angela Lauria and The Author Incubator's team, as well as to David Hancock and the Morgan James Publishing team for helping me bring this book to print.

Thank You

I am so thankful to you, my reader, for picking up this book.

It is my ultimate desire to help the Superwomen of the world lose their weight and find themselves again.

You have read this book and are on your way to weight loss and balance in your life.

Do you see yourself as the woman who goes the extra mile for her family, her job, and her home, and rarely do you stop to take care of yourself?

If this sounds like you, I have developed a video for you—as a thank you—to share with you what is causing that hated weight gain. You can find me at suesealwellness@gmail.com.

I am so lucky to be able to help woman not only lose the extra pounds they have gained, but to also help women who work so hard to find themselves again.

Please accept my free gift to assist you on your journey!

With love and light,

Sue

About the Author

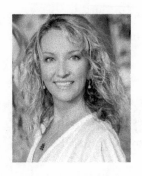

Sue Seal is an established physical therapist, an Integrative Nutrition health coach, and a Yoga-Alliance certified instructor who helps successful, hard-working women lose weight and overcome their "Superwoman" complex. During Sue's thirty years as a practicing physical therapist, she has witnessed intelligent women lose their bodies to illness and weight gain, and lose both physical strength and functional mobility of their body as they tried to juggle careers and families. Her goal is to not only help guide women to lose weight, but more importantly, to achieve greater balance in their lives.

Sue combines the Western philosophy of physical therapy with her Eastern medical beliefs, along with yoga, Jin Shin, and physical therapy, to help her clients achieve balance, harmony, and health.

Sue enjoys living in the Pacific Northwest, at her home in Bonney Lake, Washington. She graduated from the University of Puget Sound with a degree in physical therapy and received her Integrative Nutrition Health Coach certification from the Institute for Integrative Nutrition. Sue is the founder and owner of Balance Beyond the Mat, where she enjoys teaching yoga and providing a loving atmosphere for her yogis. She has been happily married for more than twenty-six years, and has two beautiful children, two dogs, Ava and Leo and her horse named Buddy.

Appendix A

Foundational Foods that Fill Our Spirit and Soul

Please rate each one of the food group on a scale of 1—10

Subject	1	2	3	4	5	6	7	8	9	10
Leisure-Time/Joy										
(Personal Growth/ Learning/Self-Developement										
Career										
Finances										
Movement/Body Work										
Home Environment										
Social Life/ Friends										
Relationship										
Spirituality										
Home Cooking										
Health: Allergies, blood pressure, gut, etcetera										

Appendix B
Adverse Childhood Experience (ACE) Questionnaire

Finding your ACE Score

While you were growing up, during your first 18 years of life:

1. *Did a parent or other adult in the household often:*
   Swear at you, insult you, put you down, or humiliate you?
   or
   Act in a way that made you afraid that you might be physically hurt?
   Yes / No
   If yes, enter 1.

2. *Did a parent or other adult in the household often:*
   Push, grab, slap, or throw something at you?
   or
   Ever hit you so hard that you had marks or were injured?
   Yes / No
   If yes, enter 1.

3. ***Did an adult or person at least 5 years older than you ever:***
   Touch or fondle you or have you touch their body in a sexual way?

   or

   Try to or actually have oral, anal, or vaginal sex with you?
   Yes / No
   If yes, enter 1.

4. ***Did you often feel that:***
   No one in your family loved you or thought you were important or special?

   or

   Your family didn't look out for each other, feel close to each other, or support each other?
   Yes / No
   If yes, enter 1.

5. ***Did you often feel that.***
   You didn't have enough to eat, had to wear dirty clothes, and had no one to protect you?

   or

   Your parents were too drunk or high to take care of you or take you to the doctor if you needed it?
   Yes / No
   If yes, enter 1

6. ***Were your parents ever separated or divorced?***
   Yes / No
   If yes, enter 1.

7. ***Was your mother or stepmother:***
   Often pushed, grabbed, slapped, or had something thrown at her?

   or

Sometimes or often kicked, bitten, hit with a fist, or hit with something hard?

or

Ever repeatedly hit over at least a few minutes or threatened with a gun or knife?

Yes / No

If yes, enter 1

8. *Did you live with anyone who was a problem drinker or alcoholic or who used street drugs?*

   Yes / No

   If yes, enter 1.

9. *Was a household member depressed or mentally ill or did a household member attempt suicide?*

   Yes / No

10. *Did a household member go to prison?*

    Yes / No

    If yes, enter 1

Now add up your "yes" answers: _____.
This is your ACE Score

Appendix C
Top Toxins to Avoid

Food list from Food Matters TV

Environmental Toxins
- Pesticides, Fungicides & Herbicides (carcinogenic)
- Fluoride (neurotoxin)
- Mercury & Lead (neurotoxin and immunosuppressant)
- EMF & EMR—Electromagnetic Frequencies and Radiation (possibly carcinogenic)
- Phthalates (hormone disruptor)

Found In: non-organic produce, tap water, amalgam fillings, mobiles, scented candles and air fresheners.

Household
- Volatile Organic Compounds (respiratory issues)
- Petroleum Solvents (damages airways)
- Formaldehyde (carcinogen)
- Butyl Cellosolve (organ damage)
- Phthalates (hormone disrupter)
- Nonylphenol

- Ethoxylates (hormone disruptor)

Found In: Non-natural cleaning products, laundry detergents and dishwasher powders.

My favorite cleaner and household products that I use are from water at Home. The cleaning supplies are not only nontoxic but they use water and the fibers of the cleaning clothes to sanitize the household. I highly encourage you to try these products out. It is the fibers in the cloth that lifts the dirt, no harmful chemicals or toxins.

http://www.myh2oathome.com/krisg

Beauty and Personal Hygiene
- Parabens (hormone disruptor)
- Sodium Lauryl Sulfate (toxicity)
- Dioxin (toxic byproduct of bleach)
- PEG Compounds (increases absorption toxins)
- Phthalates & Synthetic Fragrances (hormone disruptor)

Found In: Non-organic cosmetics, soaps, perfumes, tampons, deodorants, sanitary pads & lotions.

My favorite cleaning facial clothes again are from water at home. The cloth takes off every
single bit of mascara without any soap or oil, truly amazing.
http://www.myh2oathome.com/krisg

Packaging
- Bisphenol A (BPA) (lowers fertility)
- BPS (close to BPA) (disrupts hormones)
- Polystyrene (leaches styrene)
- Polyvinyl Chloride (breaks down into toxic chloride)
- Phthalates (hormone disruptor)

- Dioxin (carcinogen and endocrine disruptor)

Found In: plastic bottles, food storage containers & cling wrap.

I use mason jars and glass containers to hold my food prep items, never plastic.

Appendix D
Sue's Favorites

*Disclaimer: I am not being sponsored by any of these sources;
I just love them and hope you will too!*

How do you learn to enjoy cooking veggies? I was at a loss until I purchased these books:

- *Half Baked Harvest: Recipes from My Barn in the Mountains* by Tieghan Gerald
- *Hot Thai Kitchen: Demystifying Thai Cuisine with Authentic Recipes to Make at Home* by Pailin Chongchitnant
- *Six Seasons: A New Way with Vegetables* by Joshua McFadden with Martha Holmberg

(Special thanks to Bonne Holbrook for her loving guidance and selfless sharing.)

How do I cook seafood? Check out:

- *As Wild As It Gets: Duke's Secret Sustainable Seafood Recipes, Including Intimate Tales of the Legend Himself* by Duke Moscrip

To quickly learn how to add flavor to different ingredients, check out:

- *The Flavor Bible: The Essential Guide to Culinary Creativity, Based on the Wisdom of America's Most Imaginative Chefs* by Karen Page and Andrew Dornenburg

How do I clean my face and home without toxins?

- "H20 at Home" http://www.myh2oathome.com/krisg

What is my favorite nutritional journal?

- I must give credit to The Institute for Integrative Nutrition's *Daily Journal: Your Guide to a Happier, Healthier Life.*

For great mantras to use for meditation, check out:

- Heal Your Body: The Mental Causes for Physical Illness and the Metaphysical Way to Overcome Them by Louise Hays

For great online learning, check out:

- FMTV- Food Matters TV

Great website for motivation and life:

- Gabbybernstein.com

My favorite podcasts:

- *Broken Brain Podcast* with Dhru Purohit
- *Oprah's Super Soul Conversations* with Oprah Winfrey
- *Oprah's Master Class* with Oprah Winfrey
- *The Doctor's Farmacy* with Mark Hyman, M.D.

Bibliography

Amen, Daniel G. *Change Your Brain, Change Your Life: The Breakthrough Program for Conquering Anxiety, Depression, Obsessiveness, Lack of Focus, Anger, and Memory Problems.* 2nd ed., Harmony Books, 2015.

Barral, Jean-Pierre. *Understanding the Messages of Your Body: How to Interpret Physical and Emotional Signals to Achieve Optimal Health.* North Atlantic Books, 2008.

Beck, Martha. *Finding Your Own North Star: Claiming the Life You Were Meant to Live.* Three Rivers Press, 2001.

Buettner, Dan. *The Blue Zones: 9 Lessons for Living Longer From the People Who've Lived the Longest.* 2nd ed., National Geographic, 2012.

Burmeister, Alice, and Tom Monte. *The Touch of Healing: Energizing Body, Mind, and Spirit with the Art of Jin Shin Jyutsu.* Bantam Books, 1997.

Butler-Biggs, Jane, and Alison Daniels. *The Feng Shui Directory.* The Ivy Press Limited, 2000.

Doty, James R. *Into the Magic Shop: A Neurosurgeon's Quest to Discover the Mysteries of the Brain and the Secrets of the Heart.* Avery, 2016.

Hay, Louise. *Heal Your Body: The Mental Causes for Physical Illness and the Metaphysical Way to Overcome Them.* 4th ed., Hay House, 1988.

Hyman, Mark. *Broken Brain 2: The Body-Mind Connection.* Broken Brain 2, Hyman Digital, 3 Apr. 2019, brokenbrain.com/.

Korb, Alex. *The Upward Spiral: Using Neuroscience to Reverse the Course of Depression, One Small Change at a Time.* New Harbinger Publications, Inc., 2019.

Lipton, Bruce H. *The Biology of Belief: Unleashing the Power of Consciousness, Matter & Miracles.* 2nd ed., Hay House, Inc., 2016.

Lohan, Patricia. *The Happy Home: Your Guide to Creating a Happy, Healthy, Wealthy Life.* Balboa Press, 2018.

Myers, Thomas W. *Anatomy Trains: Myofascial Meridians for Manual and Movement Therapists.* Churchill Livingstone/Elsevier, 2009.

Northrup, Christine. *Women's Bodies, Women's Wisdom: Creating Physical and Emotional Health and Healing.* 4th ed., Bantam Books, 2010.

Otto, Jonathan. *Depression & Anxiety Secrets Series.* Depression, Anxiety & Dementia Secrets, Health Secrets LLC, 2019, depressionanxietyseries.com/.

Riegger-Krause, Waltraud. *Health Is in Your Hands: Jin Shin Jyutsu Practicing the Art of Self-Healing.* Upper West Side Philosophers Inc, 2014.

Tolle, Eckart. *A New Earth: Awakening to Your Life's Purpose.* 2nd ed., Penguin Books, 2016.

Wark, Chris. *Square One: Healing Cancer Coaching Program.* Chris Wark, 2017.

Wszelaki, Magdalena. *Cooking for Hormone Balance: A Proven, Practical Program with Over 125 Easy, Delicious Recipes to Boost Energy and Mood, Lower Inflammation, Gain Strength, and Restore a Healthy Weight.* HarperOne, an Imprint of HarperCollins Publishers, 2018.

Zukav, Gary. *The Seat of the Soul.* Simon and Schuster, 1989.